MAR 1 3

THE DAY MY BRAIN EXPLODED

THE DAY
MY BRAIN EXPLODED

Ashok Rajamani

ALGONQUIN BOOKS OF CHAPEL HILL   2013

Published by
Algonquin Books of Chapel Hill
Post Office Box 2225
Chapel Hill, North Carolina 27515-2225

a division of
Workman Publishing
225 Varick Street
New York, New York 10014

The names and other identifying details of some
characters in this memoir have been changed to protect
individual privacy and anonymity.

Library of Congress Cataloging-in-Publication Data
Rajamani, Ashok.
The day my brain exploded / by Ashok Rajamani. — First edition.
pages; cm
ISBN 978-1-56512-997-9
1. Rajamani, Ashok — Health.   2. Brain — Hemorrhage —
Patients — Biography.   3. Brain — Wounds and injuries —
Patients — Rehabilitation — New York (State) — New
York — Biography. I. Title.
RC394.H37R37 2013
617.4810440092 — dc23
[B]   2012035412

10 9 8 7 6 5 4 3 2 1
First Edition

For my mother,

Sheila Rajamani,

the strongest person I know

"Who are you?" said the Caterpillar.
This was not an encouraging opening for a
conversation. Alice replied, rather shyly, "I—I hardly
know, Sir, just at present—at least I know who I was
when I got up this morning, but I think I must
have been changed several times since then."
—Lewis Carroll
Alice's Adventures in Wonderland, 1865

❂ ❂ ❂

That I exist is a perpetual surprise
which is life.
—Rabindranath Tagore
Stray Birds, 1916

❂ ❂ ❂

Oh my God!
—Charo
VH1's *The Surreal Life,* 2003

Contents

Author's Note   xi

Prologue: 2011   1

Cum and Precum: 2000, 1983   5

Aftermath: 2003–2004   12

Peanut Curry: 1974   24

The Day My Brain Exploded: 2000 (I)   28

Nonbloody Events of the Day: 2000 (II)   36

Grudge Match: Krisnha v. Jesus: 1974–1989   45

The Incarceration, Part One: 2000 (III)   54

Not The First Time in Jail: 1989–1992   70

The Incarceration, Part Two: 2000 (IV)   82

Formatting Ashok Version 2.0: 2000 (V)   96

Jeepers Creepers,

Where'd You Get Those Peepers: 2000 (VI)   123

AVM Wha . . . ?: 2000 (VII)   134

Drunk with Success: 1992–2000   138

Big Apple Core: 2000–2001   148

Time to Bloom: 2001   165

Just When You Thought the Worst Was Over: 2002   176

I Sing the Body Electric: 2002–Present   186

Through the Looking Glass: 2003–Present   199

Hermit Spiral: 2004   213

Lazarusness: 2004–Present   221

Brain Karma: 1974–___   232

No Pity Required, Just Fresh Breath: Present (I)   235

Becoming How the Brain Became: Present (II)   243

Acknowledgments   251

Author's Note

IT HAS BEEN SAID that all it takes is one bad day to reduce the sanest person to insanity. There's some truth to this. But the saying is not totally correct.

A bad day, to put it mildly, happened to me over a decade ago: my brain exploded. This was a detonation that affected not only my brain, but how I perceived the world around me. Yet it never reduced me to complete lunacy. Rather, it introduced me to a strength within, complete with the perseverance and dedication to live once again. I have my parents to thank for these qualities; not only did they raise me to be resilient, but also to be proud: proud of my cultural heritage, proud of my family, and proud of myself and my achievements. Fortunately, I got a strong intellect from them as well, along with a determination to succeed. All of that has kept me resolute as I struggled through the events you will learn about in this memoir.

Strength and determination are what I needed to overcome the effects of that day. It also took humor, in part anyway, to diffuse the anger and pain that I felt at what fate had handed me.

I believe that the worst part of this ongoing experience is happily behind me, and that I have a shiny new life to look forward to. True, what I went through was terrible, and true, I wasn't always patient with those around me. But I realize now, looking back, I am one of the luckiest people alive, and in telling my story I am hoping to give a voice to others who were not so fortunate.

Every day, dozens of people suffer from brain injury; many die, and many who live are able to function only at the mercy of devoted caregivers. I, on the other hand, now live on my own, moving among the rest of the world as though there was nothing truly wrong. Able also to write this book so that those who have suffered brain injury can, along with their caregivers, see how important it is to not give up. As I say, I am one of the lucky ones, and so I will spend the rest of this life I have been given in trying to make a difference.

But with a sense of humor, of course; I still cherish my sanity.

THE DAY MY BRAIN EXPLODED

Prologue: 2011

My calloused brown feet are hurting, aching in fact, here in Manhattan. I've just returned from a beginner's basic yoga class this afternoon, having walked all the way from that Upper East Side "Eastern Spiritual Center" back to my apartment downtown. It's a nearly seventy-minute walk, in this August, grade-A city scorcher. I've become malodorous and soaked with sweat. Being the vain fool that I am, today I chose to wear my weighty black leather shoes with the three-inch heels, rather than a practical pair of sneakers, or even flip-flops. On this boiling summer day, why did I want to add those extra inches of height to my mediocre five foot eight frame? Especially when I had to remove the shoes and be barefoot as soon as class began anyway? Maybe I just wanted to look tall when I entered the center so I could flirt with the instructor.

Before getting into my apartment, I had to walk up six

flights of stairs in my elevatorless building. This doesn't make matters any better.

So here I am, wet, smelly, and tired. Turning on the AC to full force and picking up my best buddy, the remote control, off the sofa, I click to find a station worthy of my sticky summer viewing.

Now, I must admit, these days, I'm a proud member of geek central. Meaning that my cable television is usually set to two types of programming: news channels with some shows featuring child predators, and science channels.

I decide to watch some nondescript science network. All I see is a black screen with lights flashing in it, set to the beat of some innocuous, gloomy orchestral music. I've just missed the title credits, so I don't know the exact name of the show, but based on the ominous music, I surmise it's one of those random programs about the history of the universe. As soon as I hear a deep, sedate voiceover, I realize I'm right. Not sure if I'm listening to James Earl Jones or Morgan Freeman or the guy who does the Geico ads. I think it's Morgan. The voice explains that, while there are many ideas about how the world was created, this show will be about science's most accepted theory: the Big Bang Theory. And though this theory has many different angles, Morgan continues, the show will focus on only one thesis—the concept that the Big Bang Theory revolves around one word:

Explosion.

Morgan's voice continues to boom. The Big Bang, he

explains, was a mammoth explosion that happened billions of years ago, and it all began as a bursting of a primeval fireball. Just listening to that opening sentence of the program leaves me spellbound, so I think I'll be viewing this take on the Big Bang. But even though the theory is not definitively proven, it rings absolutely true to me.

That's simply because, as sweat-drenched and as exhausted as I might feel at this moment, I can understand a primary truth: it only takes a solitary, single, massive explosion to create a completely new universe.

Cum and Precum: 2000, 1983

Wedding Day Orgasm 2000

Perverted. Masturbating on your older brother's wedding day is perverted, isn't it? Well then, call me a perv. Because that's what I was doing, in my hotel room, a few hours before the ceremony.

March 17, 2000. Twenty-five years old.

The day before, I had flown from New York City to Washington, D.C., where my older brother, Prakash, and his fiancée, Karmen, lived, and were to marry. At the time of my spontaneous onanism, the rest of my family was out, playing tourists. My brother Prakash was in the room next to mine, preparing for his big day.

Now, people practice the art of self-love at various times and for just as many reasons. They might be feeling randy or simply utterly bored. In my case, it was the latter. Weddings don't make me feel amorous. And so, I prepared myself for a little diversion. I hadn't yet changed into my formal wedding suit; I was wearing an outfit appropriate for a jerk-off: a ratty eighties Def Leppard tour T-shirt. Nothing else. I set myself to the task, watching my progress in the big mirror over the dresser.

As my solo act came to its usual splashy end, I felt a sudden, massive *pop* inside my head.

I had jerked off innumerable times before, but this orgasm was different; this orgasm was unnatural.

Something was wrong, horribly wrong.

I felt a fierce explosion in my head.

In a mere instant, the equivalent of an atomic bomb had been detonated within my skull. Between my ears. Behind my eyeballs.

My brain had become Hiroshima.

I suddenly could see nothing as the bomb blasted. It was as if a blindfold, making the world darker than a moonless, starless night, had been tightly bound around my head. *Oh my god,* I thought. *I'm fucking blind! That's what the explosion was. Those rumors about jerking off were right.* Had my palms also become hairy?

Within a second, however, my sight had returned, albeit faintly. Everything was hazy, as if enveloped by fog. Caught between fear and confusion, I fell to the faded hardwood floor, straining to look at the pseudo-crystal chandelier above my head.

I felt as weak as a baby, but not a baby entering this world—rather, one leaving it. My head was filled with unimaginable pain; my universe was slowly leaving me. Strange how the body knows what it knows. I *knew* I was going to die. So my survival instinct took over, and with the little strength and vision I had, I was able to locate the hotel phone. I clawed at the receiver, thrust it to my ear and painfully pushed "0." I croaked out a plea for an ambulance.

"We're right next door to the hospital," the hotel operator chirped, as if she were merely telling me where to find the nearest vending machine. "Is there anyone who could take you there? It would be quicker."

I gave her my last name, and she paged Prakash. When he answered the phone, I bet he was still fumbling with his cummerbund.

Prakash rushed next door to my hotel room and discovered me on my bed. Surprisingly, despite the brain explosion, my sense of modesty had prevailed. Through the deadly haze and the pain and the panic, I had somehow been able to slip on my Hanes briefs. My brother found me horizontal on the bed, barely lucid, my arms crossed over my chest.

It was an oddly regal pose. Prakash had now discovered his baby brother cast as a dying pharaoh atop a hotel sarcophagus, a seemingly doomed king headed somewhere other than the River Styx, wearing nothing but an eighties metal T-shirt and a pair of tighty-whiteys.

Library Lesson 1983

The library's carpet may have dampened the noise in the room, but it also dampened the spirit. This place was depressing.

The school, named Avon, like the cosmetics line, had a library that consisted of barely one floor and featured five large Rolodexes of index cards, too few to even employ the Dewey decimal system. Since this was the early eighties, there were no computers, but only five Rolodexes? Was that really all the books we needed to read?

I was eight then, and wore big black glasses that probably accounted for one quarter of my entire body mass. Otherwise I was a small, scrawny, sienna-hued skeleton of a third grader.

When I entered the book-lined space, I frowned, not because of the perennially stale odor, but because the musty brown shag transformed the library into a space that was not just uninviting, but menacing.

The shelves themselves were disjointed, with gray steel mixing with burgundy wood. There was a sense of chaos and quiet gloom about the room. But still, it was my favorite place.

I came there every day, when we had recess from one to two in the afternoon. I never entered the playground. The idea of forced recreation didn't appeal to me.

One chilly afternoon in 1983, as I was choosing my own adventure in a *Choose Your Own Adventure* book, six of my classmates barged in, ruddy from their play. Two were girls, the rest boys.

I put my book down on the plastic table at which I was seated, and watched them swarm in.

"Hey Ashok!" Jack boomed, pronouncing my name with alarming accuracy.

Jack was their leader, robust and blond, with skin the color of ketchup-meets-mayo. The other boys and girls all could have passed for his brothers and sisters, some with blond hair, some with brown, but all white, robust, and loud.

Commander Jack barked to his supplicants.

"Ashok is so brainy!"

Huh?" I was confused, but thrilled. *He thinks I'm smart!*

"I said you're brainy," he said and sneered at me.

"Thanks, Jack!" I smiled, broadly displaying what would later become pre-orthodontia buckteeth.

"That's not a good thing, jerk."

"What are you talking about? My mom calls me brainy all the time! It means she thinks I'm smart!"

"It means you're too weak to do anything but study. It mean's you're worse than a wimp."

"Nuh-uh, you're joking," I said. "It doesn't mean that!"

"It means you're not even cool enough to be a nerd or a geek!"

His cohorts started laughing as he continued his harangue.

"Every day you come here! Why don't you go outside and play?"

Renee giggled. "He's too brainy to play house with the girls, even!"

"No way," I said. "I'm not like that!"

"Brainy!" squealed Carl.

"Brainy!" squealed Leslie.

"Brainy!" squealed Rob.

I felt helpless, and suddenly terribly ashamed.

"Maybe he wets his bed, and pees when he plays!" said Leslie.

"Leave me alone!" I yelled.

I tried to defend myself. "I'm not even here to read! I just come to look at the covers!" It was a weak, weak defense, too weak to even be lame.

They snickered and were joined by five more burly kids, running in from recess. Their taunts grew louder and louder.

The mantra was awful.

"Brainy!"

It was such a harmless, ridiculous insult, but words, in the mouths of kids, mean something different. I had thought being brainy was a good thing, but it had become an insult and a taunt, upsetting enough to make me cry within a proverbial blink.

My wonderful classroom teacher, Ms. Linds, ended the

nightmare, entering the room after hearing the shouts and loud voices. In her late twenties and with shoulder-length auburn hair, she was a white Aussie transplant with a wonderful accent.

This sweet lady told the kids that recess was over, and she forced them to leave. After I explained to her what happened, she touched my shoulders and affectionately embraced my head.

She smelled of lavender.

"Why are you crying you silly thing? They were only making fun because they're jealous," said Ms. Linds.

She hugged me as my tears dried.

"Now, give me a smile and let's go back to class."

But still I felt ashamed, and no amount of cajoling would make my grimace go away.

"Ashok, remember what I'm going to tell you."

Attempting to avoid her gaze, I surveyed my tiny hands, which were now wobbling restlessly upon my lap.

"Are you listening? I said to remember this."

"Okay, okay, I'll remember," I murmured, looking up at her through my smeared glasses.

Ms. Linds' eyes met mine.

"Being brainy," she said, "is never, ever, a bad thing."

As much as I adored her, I just didn't believe her.

Aftermath: 2003–2004

Don't compare apples to oranges. All of you are in different areas in life. Remember that. Different categories completely."

Kari, the moderator and social worker of the brain injury support group, was trying to give us a pep talk.

"You need to understand that your lives changed after your brain injuries. Understand that point, and you won't get jealous or hurt," she continued.

It didn't work. Out of the twenty attendees in the room, four, including me, were still morose, sad, and bitter. I was there because everyone—neurologists, therapists, counselors—told me to join a group as soon as I was released from the hospital. But it took almost four years for me to actually attend a meeting. I had never planned to go, but finally I was so lonely and depressed that I felt I had no choice. Most of all,

I had become painfully envious of everyone around me. To live in the outside world again, I needed to cope with non-brain-injured folks, whom I called "norms" a la old-school carnival-freak patois. These norms, with their goddamn unscarred heads, were pissing me off. They would never understand what had happened to me.

I was nervous that first day as I made it to room 10B in the Center for Disability, a run-down, twelve-story building on Manhattan's Lower East Side. I had never before considered myself "disabled," but now, as I begrudgingly accepted that possibility, I tried to prepare myself for my first meeting with my new peers.

Twenty people, wearing resigned expressions, sat on cheap blue plastic folding chairs arranged in a circle. The dingy white walls, offset by blackened gray tiles on the floor, enclosed a room that was suffocating in stale air. On one wall hung a framed poster of a striped cat with a word-balloon over its head that said, "I meow, therefore I am." I imagined Descartes's reaction if he had seen this. He wouldn't have just rolled over in his grave. No, he would have climbed out, purchased a Colt .45, and shot himself.

Daunted but not deterred, I looked closer. All those in the circle displayed evidence of brain injury. Some had paralyzed legs, some were blind, some were deaf. Some were quadriplegic.

My average frame looked downright Charles Atlasesque next to some of the weakened bodies I saw before me.

This was one of the rare occasions when I didn't wear my contact lenses, so my view was slightly obscured by the scratches on the thick lenses in my Buddy Holly frames.

The glasses accentuated my fleshy nose while downsizing my large eyes, which were widening in horror as I took time to look closely at everyone gathered there.

Of course, my looks hardly mattered at that point, and I knew it was ridiculous to even contemplate how I appeared. I had entered a room where fashion was the least of anyone's concerns.

After each member had been seated, the moderator introduced herself as Kari, and welcomed us to "the once-a-month brain support session," as she called it. She was a petite, attractive mid-thirties white woman who worked at the nearby hospital as a social worker.

The room was chillingly quiet, as in support group tradition we told our stories one by one. I suddenly had monstrous pangs of guilt. I was one of the few there whose ailments, while severe, appeared nonexistent. I wasn't in a wheelchair. Though half-blind, I could see. I could hear. I could speak. And, yes, I could samba.

I had always been irritated about this lack of obvious scarring, thinking mine to be a silent disease. Nobody could look at me and tell that I had a scorched battlefield between my ears, in part because, by all accounts, my brain still worked. I could articulate my thoughts, and even better, I had thoughts to begin with.

We went around the circle, each of us sharing our circumstances. We were different ages, different races, and different genders. The one commonality was brain injury. But even our brains were altered in diverse ways. Three of the younger ones, maybe in their twenties, couldn't speak at all; they sat in wheelchairs and simply nodded.

An overweight mid-fifties white woman with an unkempt gunmetal bob sat lazily in her chair. Wearing an oversized gray running jacket over a shapeless green sweatsuit, she had a foolish grin and drooled thickly.

Kari smiled at the woman, whose name, she told us, was Sara.

"Sara's just started speaking these past few weeks," she said with pride.

Everyone smiled.

"She now can form full sentences," she said, her pride even more pronounced.

Everyone applauded.

I learned after the meeting that Sara had been living with brain injury ever since the early nineties, when she was involved in a three-car accident on the Long Island Expressway.

She was the only driver substantially injured. Kari gave me the background.

"That's terrible," I said, "but even though she's in bad shape, it's great that she's speaking again."

"I know," Kari said, "I'm so happy for her progress. Just last year, she didn't even understand the meaning of the word 'the.'"

"That's fantastic," I said, attempting a forced cheerfulness that unsuccessfully masked my sadness. "What was she doing before her injury?"

"She was a corporate lawyer."

Our group also included a former model. A brain bleed had left half of her face paralyzed. She looked like she was wearing a mask.

One distinguished-looking middle-aged black man dressed in a suit stood up. His companion, who could have been his twin, or lover, or friend, said the dapper fellow was named Matt, and had been a heart surgeon.

Matt shushed him. "I can speak for myself, Tim," he barked. "I just want to tell everyone how proud I am of myself!"

We waited for Matt to continue, but he didn't say anything more. He simply sat down again, closed his eyes, and began rubbing his face. He looked exhausted.

Tim broke the silence.

"I'm proud of him, too," he said, without revealing the

nature of Matt's injury. "Time for show-and-tell," he said and turned to his friend.

Matt revealed to us the reason for the delight: he stood up, opened his right hand, and showed us a small metallic object.

Then, like a five-year-old thrilled to understand finally the difference between a nickel and a quarter, Matt exclaimed, "For a while I've been thinking this is only some stupid pointy thingy. But now I totally understand what this is! I know what this is! It goes in your skin!"

He was holding a syringe.

A tall, attractive thirtysomething white man with long-ish black hair stood up. His companion, an elderly white woman, immediately told us the gentleman had been an es-tablished soap opera actor.

The man seemed to have come straight from a fashion shoot, decked out in sleek black slacks and a fitted blue sweater that hugged his well-built body. I wondered why a guy so sharp was in a place like this.

When he started talking, I understood.

"My-y-y-y-y- n-n-n-nayy-y—"

It took him more than a minute to utter "my name."

One of the group's main rules was not to interrupt any member when he or she was speaking. We waited out the next two minutes, until he was able to complete "My name is Charles." But his main problem was not stuttering; he seemed to be floating in and out of lucidity itself. In the next breath, he began speaking coherently, but extremely slowly. Like a three-year-old reading *Mary Had a Little Lamb*.

Even though I was curious to find out the anatomy of his injury, nobody asked him. Perhaps that was the code of the group, I figured, to let everybody speak the way they wanted to, and to tell only as much as they felt comfortable revealing.

Standing up, he recounted the day-by-day schedule of his week. Everybody listened carefully, even me. Usually I had a tendency to be impatient and interrupt. But I said nothing and joined the others in offering silent nods until he was done feeding us his datebook.

Kari picked me to follow Charles. When I was done confessing, I looked around the room. Everyone appeared shocked. One wheelchair-bound elderly Hispanic woman, who had yet to speak in group, introduced herself as Natalie.

She stared at me.

"You seem very healthy and well-spoken, young man," she said. "You must have had the brain injury around ten years ago, am I right?"

"Not really," I said, looking down.

"Oh my gosh, I'm sorry. It was probably more than ten. That was stupid of me. I know brains take a long time to recover, honey."

Her face became solemn. "Even if it's taken you fifteen years, or your whole life to recover, you should be proud. You're still alive, and that's all that matters."

"Actually," I said, "this happened to me three years ago."

"Listen, kiddo," she responded, displaying hints of irritation. "Be serious. When did you have your trauma?"

I tried to explain that I was telling the truth, but nobody in the group seemed convinced.

Then the soap star stood up again. Perhaps feeling encouraged by my openness to talk, he was ready to tell us what happened to him.

Whereas before he couldn't even speak one sentence coherently, now Charles's words came out with eerie clarity. He started slowly, and progressed to a faster pace.

"Ten years ago . . .

". . . my boyfriend was saying bye to me in the Fourteenth Street subway station at midnight waiting for the E train must have been behind a stalled car since it was taking so long to get to me. . . .

"Mike and I had been holding hands and hugged when he left I didn't think . . .

". . . much about it

"Two minutes after he left a cop comes up to me. . . . He holds his crotch and asks me if I want it. I looked shocked and as soon as I say something he punches me in the face calls me all the names you can think of . . .

"He punches me four or five more times I beg him to please stop I'll do what you want please stop he doesn't I can't think straight when he's finished he pushes me into the tracks I survived I ate pizza for breakfast today and . . . I held the slice with these many fingers"

Charles held up three fingers on his right hand.

After recounting his tale, Charles left, with his companion. The silent room became, impossibly, even quieter.

Of Hair and Heroin

After receiving increasingly upsetting stares by strangers, I let my hair grow long to cover the carved back of my skull. I refused to go to any barber, especially my former hairstylist. But one steamy, sweltering day in mid-August, I finally gave in to the heat. I wanted a haircut from him, and only him.

His name was Phil, a fortysomething Italian man with long flowing red hair and a bushy red beard. His thick, hairy arms were covered with tattoos—eagles, tigers, thunderbolts, the word *Mom*—making him look like a biker, or at least a trucker. Phil was an anomaly in the prissy, faux-manly runway world of Chelsea. Imagine the love child of Willie Nelson and Hulk Hogan—that would be Phil.

Phil asked where I'd been for so long. I told him the story. He listened silently and then exploded with a loud laugh.

"Still the same Ashok," he said, "always joking."

But as he began cutting my hair, clearing away the deep growth on the back of my head, the scar came into view. Phil gasped.

"You mean your skull was really opened?"

"Phil, bone don't lie."

Gently grabbing a handful of my hair, Phil parted the

mop again to get a full view of my skull-steel. "That is one awesome scar," he said, then whistled. Clearly he had new respect for me.

I told him to do anything that would cover the devastation and watched in the mirror as Phil examined the scar. Then he looked up, a mischievous glint in his eyes.

"Let's cut it all off."

"Are you crazy?" I whined. "The scar is disgusting. I want it totally hidden. Everybody stares and makes comments about it." I realized that I sounded like a thirteen-year-old girl.

Over my shoulder, Phil gave me a hard, deep look in the mirror.

"Do you think that veterans feel that way? That scar is a badge of honor. It means you survived."

"Oh yeah, and what the hell do you know about this kind of surviving?" I said.

His face suddenly became serious. "I know all about it," he said. "I survived a killer. Heroin."

This was news to me. *It's kinda cool*, I thought, *having a former junkie cutting my hair.*

"Twice," he said. "I was hooked for over ten years, before my wife finally pushed me into rehab. But two weeks after my release, I reunited with my true love. I became an addict all over again."

"I didn't know," I said.

"I tried everything, even methadone. No dice. After my second stint in rehab, I finally quit shooting up. Cold turkey.

"I'm not saying that I can possibly know what you went through," he quickly added. "But I know what it is to live through a nightmare."

"At least you don't have a permanent physical reminder," I said, surveying his big, furry arms for track marks. Perhaps the tattoos had covered them.

Phil sighed. "A long time before coming here to Chelsea, I ran a barbershop in Queens. Real roughneck joint. I used to cut gang members' hair. They asked me to shave designs into their flattop fade cuts, stuff like shapes, gang symbols."

My mind wandered back there, to the years before my head exploded; hearing about flattop fades made me think about eighties rap music and Adidas footwear.

"Hey Phil, remember 'Rapper's Delight'? Remember when hip-hop first came out?"

He sighed, obviously irritated by my lack of attention. In turn, he ignored my question. "These guys would have paid to have your scar. It's hardcore. Looks like the Batman logo without the bat. And without the oval."

I laughed. By comparing me to Bruce Wayne's alter ego, he won me over. I let Phil shave my head completely. When he finished, he turned me around and held a mirror behind my head so I could see what I had been hiding under my hair.

Butchered. My head was butchered. Yet as I scrutinized the back of my skull, for the first time I felt no shame.

"Be proud, Ashok. You're like a POW. If anyone asks you about the scarring," he said with a chuckle, "say you got it in a war!"

Smiling broadly now, I paid for the trim and gave Phil a big tip.

Phil may have been kidding when he made that remark, but he was right.

It was a war all along.

Peanut Curry: 1974

Fuck Holden Caulfield or David Copperfield or any other overanalyzed fictional white guy.

Let's talk about an Indian American guy for once, a nonfictional brown guy who Mr. Caulfield would likely walk past, even if he saw the brown guy getting bashed by a gang of white supremacists in a dark alley.

And let's begin by discussing how the brown guy had once been Baby Buddha.

"Once upon a time," my mother would tell me as a child, "there was a pretty Indian woman. She loved eating peanuts all the time. So she gave birth to a peanut."

Okay, so she never actually told me that fairy tale, but I was, indeed, called Peanut by the nurses who helped her give birth to me in 1974, in a tiny hospital in New Brunswick, New Jersey.

This was the real tale told by my mom, a slender and petite South Indian woman named Sheila. With a complexion of deep, rich cocoa, she had fleshy cheeks and thick, waist-length hair, usually tied in a loose, braided ponytail. Her large, chocolate almond-shaped eyes shone under meticulously plucked, arched eyebrows.

At twenty-five, barely measuring five foot four and a little over one hundred pounds, she was already mother to Prakash, born three years earlier.

Expecting her second baby in early December of 1974, she was astonished to awake with contractions on the morning of November 3, at around ten o'clock. Even though it wasn't too early in the morning, it was a Sunday, the day of the week on which my parents would usually sleep until noon. But no such luck on this day. Sunday morning or not, I was up and ready to go.

"It's time," she whispered to my father, who had been snoring loudly and peacefully. His slim five-foot-eight frame was wrapped in a flimsy white T-shirt and his standard dhoti, the south Indian male sarong, which resembled a transparent, floorlength white skirt.

Mahogany-hued with an oversized honker that I would inherit, his name was Rajamani. His full moniker was Puthucode Narayanswamy Rajamani, the first name being the town of his birth, the second being the name of his father, and the third being his actual birth name. This was the custom of our people, South Indian Tamil Palghat Brahmins. Technically, then, his name was simply Rajamani. Like Cher. He called himself Raj.

Upon awakening, he responded groggily. "You're just having gas, Sheel; we have another whole month until the big day. Go back to sleep."

She responded by turning on the light.

In just a few minutes, Mom and Dad and a sleepy Prakash were on the way to the nearest hospital in Dad's beatup blue Chevy Vega.

After quickly signing the paperwork at the front desk, Mom told Dad to take Prakash, who was screeching at the top of his lungs, to the home of their friends, Shrini and Thangam, a cheery married couple. Dad resisted at first but eventually yielded.

Left in the care of the nurse, Mom was wheeled to her room, where she practiced her Lamaze techniques, hoping her husband would return quickly.

By the time he returned, just forty minutes later, I had been born. It was right before noon.

Dad yelled joyfully when he was told Mom had given birth to another son.

By the time he arrived, I had already been given a nickname. Since I was born prematurely, almost an entire five weeks before the standard nine-month pregnancy delivery date, I weighed barely five pounds.

The doctor and nurses called me "Peanut."

I was not crying. I was wrinkly, dusky, and oddly serene, with East Asian eyes. And because I was dark, the total effect was that of a Southeast Asian newborn.

An ancient Tibetan, if you will. The doctor even jokingly asked Mom if the Dalai Lama was the father.

So Peanut was given an extra nickname: Baby Buddha.

The real name my parents gave me, of course, was neither. But they chose it precisely because of my placid demeanor: *Ashok*, in Sanskrit, means "one without sorrow."

The Day My Brain Exploded: 2000 (I)

The Discovery

Time seemed to blaze through a blackened stretch of un-discovered galaxies following my hotel room collapse. When my eyes opened, and clear sight had finally returned, I had no idea where I was.

Fuck Fuck Fuck.

I was in a bed. But where? I looked up. High above me, a metallic, gray-steel ceiling spread out overhead. Then I saw Prakash's face staring down at me, a terrible mingling of fright, anxiety, and terror.

This didn't look good at all.

"You're in a hospital," he said. "They say you've had a brain hemorrhage. Your brain bled."

No way. There was no blood. Just some cum.

"You're in a hospital," he repeated when he saw my look

of horror. "You don't remember? I picked you up a while ago from the hotel room and walked you here. You've been pretty much unconscious, sleeping since I got you here. The doctors just took a CT scan of your head."

I then noticed Mom standing next to Prakash.

Both were silent. Next to them stood a pink-faced man in a white coat. Extremely skinny, balding, and sporting a scraggly white beard, he looked like an anorexic Santa Claus.

"Ashok, I'm Dr. Brown. You gave us quite a scare. Let me tell you what happened."

"Prakash told me I had a brain hemorrhage," I said.

"Yes, you did. It's called a Subarachnoid Intracranial Cerebral Hemorrhage, and after taking the CT scan, we discovered the cause of it," he continued, holding out an X-ray in front of my face.

He pointed to a major dark spot on the bottom left corner of the brain scan. I inspected it. Prakash and Mom moved in closer for a better look.

"See that?" he said.

We all nodded.

"That," he said, "is an AVM. AVM means Arteriovenous Malformation. I assume you've never heard that term."

Even in my blurry state, I almost replied sarcastically, out of habit, "Duh."

"An AVM is a tangle of veins and arteries hidden in the brain," he explained.

Prakash suddenly lashed out at me. "See what you get for all your whacking off?" Clearly I must have told him about my private activity before the wedding, although I couldn't remember doing it. Mom's face contorted into a grim, stony-faced mask, looking as though her tightened, immobile lips would prevent her from bursting into a flood of tears.

"An AVM is not caused by anything," Dr. Santanorexic said quietly. "It is a congenital birth defect—a defect that develops in the fetus during the third month of pregnancy. Behavior didn't cause it. Ashok was born with it.

"The AVM hemorrhage was going to happen someday— turns out today was the day. It usually bursts in a person between the ages of twenty and forty. Many brain hemor-rhages and aneurysms are urogenitally based, meaning that they usually happen when a person's having sex, giving birth, going to the bathroom. In your case, your brother told me you were masturbating."

He turned to me. "The second you orgasmed, your blood rushed to the brain with severe pressure. The AVM ruptured because of it, causing your brain to bleed, flooding your head with septic fluid. Ashok, AVM bleeds can be fatal."

He then looked at my family and said gravely, "It's a won-der he's still here."

The fog in my head scattered with this new information. So this disgusting tangle had been hiding in my brain since I was in Mom's womb. It was my inheritance: a murderous genetic inheritance.

One would think this news to be the perfect antidote to Prakash's scolding, the medical information to absolve me of any responsibility. But deep down, I still believed I was at fault. I had been bad, playing with myself on my brother's wedding day. I had caused the hemorrhage. But, of course, I hadn't.

Pre-explosion

Oddly enough, I was able to regain consciousness temporarily. Much later, I found out through a neurologist that most people who suffer brain hemorrhages fall into unconsciousness briefly after their explosion, then return to lucidity for a few hours, and then lose it once again.

This would explain how I could later remember assessing the enormity and seriousness of what had happened, while at the same time recalling bits of my life leading to the bleed—namely, my home, which at the time was a huge top-level Chelsea studio apartment, complete with fireplace.

My job in public relations was quite lucrative, which was why I could afford such an apartment. I loved that flat of mine. A major problem, however, was my insurance. I had just recently left one job and taken a higher-level position at another public relations firm—but that was just a week or so before my explosion. Which meant I had no health insurance from the new company yet, as they only doled that out some months after employment commenced. Which meant I was left to rely on the COBRA insurance

from my earlier job. The only problem: I didn't recall signing the COBRA form.

Though awake, as my lucidity began its disappearing act,
I was still unable to absorb the reality of it all. Everything
seemed to be in slow motion as Prakash, Mom, and I looked
at each other in silence. Then Dad entered the room, visibly
angry, his thinning hair askew, gray plastic glasses nearly falling off his sweat-soaked face.

"What's happening with your insurance?" he demanded.
There it was, the insurance issue. I knew it was a problem,
but had no idea how it would affect me so much at that exact
time—in the midst of my brain bleeding away.

"Huh?" I said to Dad, my head still aching fiercely. I
couldn't believe I was being interrogated.

"I just called your former employer. The goddamn office
manager informed me that you never signed your COBRA
insurance form when you left. You had sixty days, you moron. Now we might have to pay millions just to keep you
alive!"

"Dad, are you psycho?" Prakash intervened. "Ashok could
die any moment!"

Mom said nothing, her round moon-face wilting. Not
yet changed for the wedding, she was wearing her faded
jeans and loose gray sweater. Her lush black hair was untied,
messily falling around her shoulders. Her face was without
makeup, the dark brown skin naked as she began crying

softly. Mom's Estée Lauder eggplant lipstick—her cosmetic trademark—had been smudged away.

"Have common sense," Dad replied in a voice betraying an equal mixture of anger and fear. "This *will* be his deathbed if we can't afford to keep him alive. Insurance is all that matters at this point."

Prakash, Mom, and even the doctors appeared stunned at Dad's outburst. Moments after having my brain detonate, I was having another medical emergency: I was being ripped a new asshole.

Luckily, Prakash was an attorney. He quickly called the office manager for my old employer and insisted that I was still entitled to full insurance even though I hadn't signed off. After much arguing between them, she finally agreed. I was saved.

I looked with gratitude at my big brother. Prakash, over six feet tall and skinny, was still in his tuxedo slacks. His long-sleeved dress shirt was now unbuttoned, wrinkled and sweat-stained.

The last few hours had aged him beyond his twenty-eight years. His chiseled face was pale and looked downright skeletal. His eyes were swollen and dark.

But his hard work on the phone paid off. Now that I was insured, Dad could breathe again, safe in the knowledge that his bank account wouldn't be emptied.

• • •

Hell Begins

Immediately after dealing with the insurance debacle, the real nightmare started. Thoughts churned wildly in my damaged mind as the effects of the explosion made their way through my body. All I really understood was that I was losing my freedom to move. I later learned that, right at this moment, my exploded brain had exposed my body to a tidal wave of murderous bacteria. I was moved immediately from the ER to the Intensive Care Unit.

Though unaware of my actions, I had become hysterical from the hemorrhage, and like an animal caught in an unforgiving trap, I tried to pull my arms free of the IV pole, and tried to kick myself off the bed. The doctors were forced to strap me in.

I began burning with a high fever and started vomiting. And as the raw torture caused my consciousness to slowly descend into delirium, my earlier shocks of confusion were lessening, transforming into horror and fear.

My insides felt scalded, with the shockwaves brought on by the hemorrhage unleashing too much radiated heat for my body to handle. The pain caused my damaged brain to shut down; I felt my mind rapidly slipping away. The doctors then decided to administer a spinal tap to check the amount of noxious blood and fluid swirling inside me.

I sensed my head being split apart, the middle a bloody yolk. My torn brain was continuing to spill itself into me, flooding my internal organs with an excess of unhealthy cerebrospinal fluid, or CSF.

Another CT scan was performed. While it showed no new complications, this was little consolation; CSF continued its deadly flow throughout my brain.

I sensed I was now bypassing purgatory and going straight into the lake of fire.

Nonbloody Events of the Day: 2000 (II)

Spanking my monkey into a brain-bleed, of course, was not how the wedding day had begun.

When I first arrived in D.C., on Thursday, I had not felt well. My throat hurt, my nose dripped, my ears ached. Everyone else was excited about the nuptials—but I only felt miserable. I went to a nearby pharmacy, bought some over-the-counter cold syrup, and hoped for the best.

The wedding was set for the next day at 5 p.m. But when I awoke that morning, there was little change in my condition. As the others headed downstairs to the hotel restaurant for breakfast, I begged off and stayed in my room. I told them I still felt ill.

Most of our family—aunts, grandparents, cousins, et cetera—lived in India. Here in America, we only had a couple of uncles.

Our blood representatives for the marriage, then, were few. Only my mother's brother, Sunil Uncle, and his two-year-old daughter, Supriya, had come for the wedding. For most people, having so little family in attendance might be depressing, but we were grateful just to have these two. Like abandoned children in an unvisited neighborhood, my small family—Dad, Mom, Prakash, and I—had been alone in America throughout our lives.

After breakfast, the five came upstairs to my room with plans to tour D.C. They would take a trolley to the White House, the Lincoln Monument, the Smithsonian, and the Arlington National Ceremony. My father had it all planned. I just shrugged. I still felt like shit and was going to sleep in.

Prakash and Karmen, his bride-to-be, were delighted that the family was leaving. After all, they had their own plans: Prakash wanted to hang with his *boyz* around the hotel; Karmen wanted to have a "beauty" day: spa treatment, massage, and skin pampering. She would meet up later with her dad and brother who had flown in from Florida.

Months after my hospitalization, Mom dutifully described to me the events of that unimaginable day. It was an especially chilly day, unusual even for March. The group left the hotel at 10 a.m. with Dad determined to see as much as he could. I learned later that he kept everyone on the tour despite the cold—even though Supriya, unaccustomed to the frigid weather, was clearly uncomfortable. When Mom asked that they return to the hotel, Dad brushed her off.

"The next stop is Arlington Cemetery," he said with fervor. "We can't miss it, I've heard so much about it."

"Why are you so obsessed with that place? Supriya's not feeling well. Let's go back."

Only after they had walked through the miles of monuments and acres of white stone crosses did Dad finally give in. At 3 p.m., they returned to the hotel.

Upon reaching the hotel room all four were sharing, the first thing they noticed was the telephone. Its red light was blinking furiously, insistently, as though it was caught in a seizure. The answering machine display read twenty-five messages. Dad quickly punched the PLAY button.

"Come quick," Prakash shrieked. "Ashok is in the hospital!"

That was followed by: "Ashok is in the ER, he had an aneurysm, *Oh my God!*"

The next twenty-three messages were variations of the first two, each transmitted in Prakash's most frantic voice.

After discovering that Dad's cell phone had been off during the entire tour, Mom turned on him, her eyes blazing.

"How could you waste time in the goddamn cemetery?!" she screamed. "How could you be so oblivious and not turn on your cell phone?!"

Dad didn't respond, but simply opened the door and

raced out into the hall. The others followed him downstairs, through the hotel lobby and next door to the hospital. They found me in the emergency room, lying in a bed, Prakash watching over me.

Sari Bride

This was not to be Prakash and Karmen's only wedding ceremony; after all, Karmen was a devout Christian and Prakash a Hindu.

The authentic Hindu ceremony was held the day before in a temple in Maryland. Nevertheless, for most invitees, this Christian, All-American hotel version was still considered the "official" ceremony.

The Hindu ceremony had come off perfectly. Karmen was the daughter of a Filipino mother—who had passed away years before—and a white father. Genetically, it was a lovely combination. In traditional Indian bride fashion, her dark-chocolate hair was parted down the middle, and tightly knotted in a heavy, stupa-formed bun. She was quite tall, nearly matching my brother's six-foot frame.

Karmen had adorned herself in an extravagant red sari with gold border. On her forehead was a circle of brilliant crimson powder to signify her entry into wifehood. Rich red henna had been elaborately painted on her bare feet.

After Prakash placed the holy wedding necklace, the *mangal sutra*, around her neck, Karmen clasped hands with him. A priest stood before them. They took seven steps around the sacred fire, symbolizing their commitment, respect, and honor for each other. Prakash and Karmen chanted holy mantras, and the ritual was completed. No wank-induced brain-bleed disrupted the happily-ever-after scene. Not that day.

The Wedding

The big event was less than two hours following my untimely orgasm, but once I reached the hospital, it was clear I wasn't going anywhere. Sunil Uncle and Supriya had just joined Dad, Mom, and Prakash by my ER bed.

Mom was in a hellish bind: attend the wedding of her older son or stay with her younger son as he fought for his life?

She turned frantically to the doctor, wailing, "What am I supposed to do? My son's wedding is about to take place!"

"Ma'am, no need to worry," he responded calmly. "Go to your son's ceremony. We will take care of Ashok."

Mom was now sobbing uncontrollably, forced into making her own Sophie's Choice. She shook her head no.

"Ma'am, I promise you that everything will be fine. Ashok is perfectly stabilized at this point, trust me. Absolutely nothing can happen to him right now, especially in the next few hours."

"I'll be back in half an hour," she promised. She prepared to leave, full of guilt.

I closed my eyes and fell asleep.

Prakash had delayed telling Karmen of the emergency; she was still relaxing in her hotel room. When he called to explain about my hemorrhage, his bride-to-be started crying. Prakash was suddenly unsure whether to go ahead with the ceremony.

Mom had been standing next to him, and she quickly grabbed the phone.

"Karmen," she said. "This is Mother. Ashok will be fine, stay calm."

"No, he won't," she yelled. "Ashok is dying! Getting married is the least of our worries. . . . I won't do it!"

Mom barked back, "You're going to get married! You're the one who has to be strong for Prakash!"

She handed the phone back to her son. "Trust me," she told him. "It's going to be difficult, true. But your brother will be okay. This wedding will go on as planned. After all, Karmen is wearing Vera Wang" — she paused for emphasis — "and it's not a rental! Think of the eighty guests!"

That was Mom, always Martha Stewart, even if her baby was dying. Of course, Karmen and Prakash caved in. As we Rajamani men know, Mom always gets her way.

Mom ordered Prakash, Supriya, and Sunil Uncle to head back to the hotel, as she and Dad turned to the task of informing their friends who had come for the wedding: three married couples, all from America's India Central — the tri-state area — who were staying in a hotel down the road. They were our "aunts" and "uncles," terms of endearment often used by Indians to address elders. The three couples were instructed to gather in one room where they were joined by Dad and Mom.

While Dad drank a glass of water to steady his nerves, Mom explained about my brain pop. Their friends all gasped in unison, but she quickly added that the wedding would continue as planned. They all knew better than to argue with her.

"How can we help? We'll do anything," Sunita Aunty said.

"Just do one thing," Mom said. She looked all of them in the eye, one by one. "I won't be there for the reception. Promise me you'll act like surrogate parents and keep Prakash and Karmen in an upbeat mood."

They all nodded.

At that point, Dad got up and announced, "I will be missing the reception, too. I have to be there for Ashok."

"Absolutely not," Mom responded angrily. "Prakash needs at least one parent, and you'll be there to support him."

At 4:30 p.m., the wedding was about to begin. Mom and Dad changed clothes. Dad wore his tuxedo. Mom emerged wearing a grand violet-red gold-brocaded sari made of Kanjeevaram silk, India's most luxurious sari material.

And her eggplant lipstick was back on.

They went down to the lobby to join all of the guests. Later they told me of the day's events.

The wedding room was lush and romantic, and the ceremony was held in a gorgeous gazebo in the hotel's largest ballroom.

Prakash entered the room with Mom and Dad, seating them in the front row. His dress shirt had been reironed. He stood inside the gazebo, flanked only by the minister—an orthodox, silver-haired Catholic priest.

Prakash's best man was not at his side today, but lying in a hospital bed next door.

At long last, Karmen entered, walking down the aisle in her Vera Wang with her father, a naval officer, at her side. The ivory gown had a perfectly fitted square-necked, sleeveless bodice and a flowing full-length skirt.

The minister performed the routine ceremony, reciting the typical Christian ceremonial speech: "Dearly beloved yada yada I now pronounce you yada yada."

Besides the immediate family and the aunties and uncles, no one knew that I was lying in a hospital bed next door. Prakash had decided not to say anything, and most guests at the reception weren't close enough to the family to ask where I was. When I found out later, I was surprised: I would have thought they would ask. Then again, tact and I have always been strangers. At the reception, however, a couple of guests finally asked the obvious.

"Where's your mom anyway? And your brother? Why couldn't they be here?"

"They couldn't make it," was Prakash's blunt answer. Simple, yet stern enough to prevent any further dialogue on the subject.

As she had promised, Mom had left right after the wedding ceremony. When she arrived at the hospital, the sari was gone. Hello, jeans and a sweatshirt. By the time she appeared at my bed, the signature eggplant lipstick had again rubbed off completely.

Grudge Match: Krishna v. Jesus: 1974–1989

My parents are both from India, having come to the States in 1968 from Mumbai, then known as Bombay. When I was one, Dad wanted to go back to India. He packed up everything, wife, kids, and possessions, and he left America's suburban sanctuary of Indian restaurants and *desi* neighborhoods. But in returning to the motherland, Dad wasn't greeted the way he expected. Despite an MS in biochemistry, nobody would hire him.

Mom's father—quite wealthy, the president of Mumbai's biggest electricity corporation—offered to take care of our family. Dad, insistent upon his self-respect, firmly turned down his proposal and scoured the city streets for a possible job. He looked at labs, hospitals, research centers. He was rejected by all of them. At the end of a three-month, dead-end job hunt, Dad decided to return to America for good. However, his old New Jersey job was gone, and no other plants were hiring at the time. A headhunter eventually found him a job in a pharmaceutical company in Deerfield, Illinois, a suburb near the heart of Chicago.

We, however, lived in the cornfieldy village of Grayslake, which was firmly situated in the buckle of the Bible Belt. Barely considered a suburb, it was, at the time, a rundown, right-wing Christian fundamentalist Midwestern town, far from Chicago. Pat Robertson would have considered it Eden. We found a townhouse in a low-income development, Quail Creek, and lived there for sixteen years. Since Deerfield was just outside of Chicago, we could easily have lived in Devon Avenue, the city's Indian neighborhood, but my father was adamant we stay in Grayslake.

As a result, we were the only Indians there. In fact, the Rajamanis, along with one Mexican family and one black family, were the only nonwhite clans in town. And though I was, of course, aware of my somewhat different appearance, I was raised to be proud of who I was as well as of my cultural heritage, something that occasionally created a bit of tension in that environment.

I had to go to Avon Center School. Not too painful. The main problem was my name. Realistically, "Ashok" is only two syllables; it shouldn't be a problem. But on the first day of every school year, the teacher found a new, more inventive way to fuck up my name.

Some variations included *Uh-Sheek, Ah-Shook, Ass-Hock.* Even my classmates were sick of it. With a collective yell at the teacher on the first day of the school year, they would clarify: "It's UH-SHOKE!"

The new teacher, flushed with embarrassment, would then say it correctly. By the next day, though, it would be forgotten and we would start all over.

It's funny how young kids lack an instinct for racism. My skin color was not an issue. Sure, I'd be asked by a classmate, "How come you're not pink like me?" But then I'd explain my Indian background. They might not understand, but they accepted the answer. The only other person of color in elementary school was Lucy Davis, a member of the only black family in town. Though we never became close friends, the looks in our eyes showed our connection.

We felt that bond even more during the seasons we were supposed to make Christmas cards. In first grade, our teacher was a Latina named Ms. Marquez. The kids tried to depict her in their cards. As they did, one after the other called out, "She's not our color!" They held up the peach-colored crayons, which the box had conveniently labeled as "Flesh."

"We can't use Flesh color to draw her!" they exclaimed. So they used the black crayon from their boxes.

By 1985, when I was in fifth grade, Dad had gained a hefty forty extra pounds since welcoming me to the world. Mom retained her slender figure. Her biggest physical change was that she had she had chopped her ebony waist-length locks and wore her hair shoulder-length.

During that year, for classroom show-and-tell, she once made me take a small bronze statue of a Hindu deity, one of those ten-cent figurines found in any Indian knick-knack store.

I had already seen artwork and sculptures of Hindu gods and goddesses, especially Lord Krishna, with his serene, blue-skinned face, peacock-adorned hair, and golden robes. He could be seen on paintings and wall hangings in my house as well as in Indian stores and the homes of my parents' friends.

The statue I was bringing to school was of Lord Krishna as the Vishwaroopa, his multiheaded, twenty-armed avatar, representing God as the ultimate power that controlled the creation, preservation, and destruction of existence itself.

Of course, I did not know how to articulate all that at the age of ten, so Mom explained it to me in understandable terms.

"Why does he look like that, Mom?" I had asked the day earlier, confused by Krishna's multilimbed appearance.

"All of his arms and heads equal all the people in the world," she said. "It means that God is everywhere."

"So is that statue God?"

"Not exactly," she said with a chuckle. "It just shows what God means. But it's still holy."

So I brought the idol in, excited to describe this unique figure to my class.

Ms. Swenton, a fifty-year-old white woman who excelled in frumpiness, introduced me.

"Ashok is next," she said, her needle-thin, unpainted lips in action, "to show what he brought. Everyone pay attention."

Just before me, a boy showed us his pet puppy, a golden retriever named Demon. The class, of course, loved his presentation, their "oohs" and "aahs" flooding the small yellow-tiled room. It was a tough act to follow.

I went to the front, gussied up in my au courant gray turtleneck and plaid pants chosen by Mom. I looked too smokin' for Grayslake.

"Everyone," I said, "this is Lord Krishna."

The kids, still panting over Demon, shut up and listened. They seemed intrigued.

I had my speech prepared.

"He's God and this—"

Before I could continue, Leslie interrupted, her blonde pigtails bouncing.

"Ewww! You mean your God is metal? That's dumb!"

"Jesus is a man!" said Mike, who looked like a sweet, cute version of Curly from the Three Stooges.

"You should love Jesus!" some other classmates boomed.

"How stupid!" Leslie snickered. "How can God be for show-and-tell?"

The whole situation was frustrating, as I, myself, was still confused about my religion, not completely understanding that idols were not actual Gods but just symbols of one monolithic divine force.

I did know one thing, though. The Lord Krishna I was holding had many, many arms.

"Here's what's stupid," I said. "You think your Jesus is great. I've seen pictures. He only has two arms. My God has so many arms he can kick your stupid God's butt!"

I had unlocked the door to an invisible sports stadium. Three of the kids, as though rooting for one of the teams in a football game, started cheering, "Jesus! Jesus! Jesus!"

"Krishna! Krishna! Krishna!" I countered, trying to yell above the impromptu pep rally. "You know my God can beat up yours!"

Here I was, starting a holy war in elementary school. All of the white Christian children were squawking at this point.

Ms. Swenton intervened: "Okay, class, simmer down."

So the battle had to stop, forcing a draw between Jesus and Krishna.

"Time for morning break," she said.

I'M TOLD THAT when Prakash was born, he was as fair as I was dark, so while the doctors thought I looked Tibetan, they thought he looked Israeli. All these descriptions irritated my mother, who was aching to see at least one of her newborns resemble her husband.

While I loathed our small, conservative Midwestern town, Prakash loved it, enjoying everything Americana, from barbeques to the National Football League. He watched wrestling entertainment events featuring the likes of Hulk Hogan. I, however, wanted to watch *The Rocky Horror Picture Show*. Our family, of course, went to view bombastic wrestlers rather than see sweet transvestites.

Ethnic minorities in America, I once heard, adjust to white life in two ways: either by assimilating or flat-out rejecting it. Prakash chose the former.

Even from the start, we contrasted. He was a typical toddler, loud, hyperactive, and overanimated, bouncing from one place to the next. Just as my nickname of "Baby Buddha" suggested, I was sluggish and quiet, firmly immobile in my crib. Perhaps my brain's hidden tenant was already sapping vital energy. Or perhaps I was just too lazy to bother, preferring to sit and drool rather than run and yell.

Prakash's valor on his wedding day was not the first time he rescued me.

When I was an infant, he was already my savior. Mom loved to tell me how he would don her white apron as a cape while swirling round my crib, enacting the role of superhero.

Of course, he always succeeded in making me laugh, and apparently was the only one who did, as my round, glum face hardly ever smiled. When he saw me looking bored, he would take red markers and draw circles all over the white wall in front of my crib.

As we grew up, the most fun we had as young brown hicks was our time together at the Lake County Fair, a yearly festival in the county to which Grayslake belonged.

At every food stall we visited, Prakash and I would always encounter the same question and engage in the same conversation with the animated men and women behind the tables:

"Can you two boys speak English?"

At eight, when I tried to respond, "Yes!" my eleven-year-old brother would shush me.

Looking at the vendor, who was usually either a pasty white woman with a crispy-banged bouffant or a pasty white man with a crispy mullet, Prakash would shake his head sadly.

"No, we don't know the English," he said in the thickest, juiciest, messiest Indian accent possible. "Can you help us?"

"Oh that's what I thought," the vendor would say mournfully. "You poor, poor things. Have these snow cones, on the house. Just go home and try to learn our language, I'm sure you can do it."

Prakash would grab the snow cones as we walked away, always saying the same thing: "What a douchebag."

We relished the freak houses and games, gobbling all

the corn dogs we could eat. One year, when I was nine, his saviordom reached its apex. After enduring the relentless stares of all the bearded truck drivers and other folks who could squish our tiny burnt umber bodies with their thick, white fists, he finally walked through the crowd to the Ferris wheel, yelling all the way.

"Peek-A-Boo! Peek-A-Boo!"

He covered his eyes as though he were a severely mentally challenged infant. The fair-goers would stare no longer but just look away, shake their head in pity, or just talk amongst each other about those "poor ignorant injuns."

Prakash didn't realize it, but his peek-a-boo performance was flat-out avant-garde protest art at its finest.

Years later, when I was twenty-one, and living in New York City, my parents finally moved out of Illinois, to, of all places, New Jersey, the ethnic soup in which I was born.

They even moved to an area one hour from the same town where Peanut made his debut. Dad had been offered a job he couldn't refuse—and this job was located in Manhattan. It was confounding that it took almost two decades for them to move out of the Bible Belt and, when they did, that they would be living right next door to where I had run off to. But, as I would discover later, the term *confounding* would be no stranger to a description of my life.

The Incarceration, Part One: 2000 (III)

Frontal: Choke on Dry Tears

My long hospitalization was beginning as my time in the ER was ending. The first step to retain control of the excessive blood and toxic fluid expelled from the hemorrhage was a procedure called a ventriculostomy, an operation in which they drill holes in the skull and insert tiny plastic tubes, also called ventrics, to drain the fluid. The tubes were surgically pierced into my skull, sticking to my bone — ancient, jagged, and fossilized armor for the rotted wetness inside. My brain had become, simply, a liquid mess.

The ventrics inserted, my body was pumped with IV bags full of drugs to sedate me and control the increasing pain. Once I was fully stabilized, the doctors gave my family some good news: They informed my family that I was lucky — the AVM was located in the right side of the back of my brain,

a relatively safe place. But it was in the occipital lobe, the vision center.

There was more news. As a result of the bleed, I had de-
veloped meningitis. That alone could kill me.

For seventy days to follow, seventy seemingly endless days,
I fought against both the meningitis and the septic consequences of the brain fluid. Most days I was unconscious,
babbling away. On other days, I could only put forth a sem-
blance of lucidity before falling into a comalike sleep. Every
day my body was immersed in harsh drugs, including co-
deine, valium, cerebroantibiotics, and amphetamines.

Soon, the doctors had to decide how to deal with the
remnants of the AVM explosion. They consulted with my
family. There were options. Embolization meant applying
glue to the AVM to control it. Radiation would burn away
the AVM. But in both procedures, there was a strong like-
lihood that I would face another hemorrhage. The surest
solution was also the riskiest: the last option, a craniotomy.
My parents listened and decided on this, open-brain surgery.

Among the risks? Blindness, deafness, and even total paralysis. I could become a quadriplegic or a vegetable. Death
always remained the other possibility.

Luckily, we had Prithvi, a distant relative in Canada—very
distant, the uncle of a cousin of an uncle, I think—who
was a neurologist. My parents contacted him immediately,
and even though he barely knew us, he became their guide

throughout the hospitalization, dispensing advice regarding the surgery, the medications, and everything else.

As I began my long hospitalization, Dad dropped off Sunil Uncle and Supriya at the airport. Mom went to Prakash and Karmen's apartment, where she would live during my hospital stay. She saw packed suitcases; the two were to have spent their honeymoon in Fiji. The suitcases would now be unpacked.

Corpus: Count 'em, There's Two

In addition to the meningitis discovered in my immediate hospitalization, I was soon diagnosed with a second case of bacterial meningitis—a very rare type. It was discovered as the doctors noticed heightened swelling in my brain—swelling that didn't correspond with the hemorrhaging. Also, my white blood cell count was increasing rapidly.

While the first type of meningitis discovered was "staph" meningitis—a relatively common type of bacteria—the second type was a complete puzzle. Staff from the National Institute of Health (NIH) and the Center for Disease Control (CDC) came to investigate. The hospital's infectious disease doctors became a permanent fixture at my bedside.

After weeks of blood work and lab tests, including routine tests for cancer and HIV, they found the answer to one of the mysteries: meningitis due to campylobacter.

According to CDC, this ultrarare killer affected less than

1 percent of the population worldwide. It was prevalent in the Third World, originating mostly from, of all things, diseased poultry.

When I was lucid enough to think back to the days before the wedding, which seemed like centuries, I remembered ordering garlic chicken from a Chinese restaurant in Manhattan. Unwittingly, of course, but still reprehensibly, they'd quite possibly been an accomplice in the attack on my brain.

Parietal: Hallucinate

I died for your sins. I am the body of love. Find salvation through my pain.

These words, of course, connect to Christ, but for some reason I yelled them while in the hospital—and I'm not any shade of Christian. They broke loose as my mind unleashed a torrent of fictions, all of which at the time I deeply, desperately, believed. My Savior complex, I later found, was a textbook reaction. Many brain patients, especially those surviving a hemorrhage, aneurysm, or stroke, don't question the veracity of their hallucinations. My imaginary beliefs were far from imaginary to me.

The Christ incarnation was just one of many guises as my brain continued to bleed. The surgeons patiently waited for a clot to form, so they could begin planning for my craniotomy.

While they were waiting to open the jar that was my skull, my mind kept on chugging. I suffered a form of mind-rape;

my thoughts and feelings were presented nakedly, vulnerably to the world. With my brain torn and bloody, my superego had vanished. Without mental inhibition, my entire inner world, once a lush, fenced garden, had been violently laid open.

I never shut up. Sometimes the words were coherent, sometimes not. The doctors told my family to be prepared for my shifting intellect, saying that brain-injury patients travel in and out of lucidity, swimming in and out of consciousness on a daily basis. Through my incessant yelping, I was able to convey what I was feeling and seeing—primarily my hallucinations. For three months I remained in that state, existing not only in the quiet world of the Neuro-critical Care Unit, but also in the deep, dark world of my mind. Days bled into nights, nights into weeks. I had lost track of time while my entire world lay in my skull. The NCCU staff would continuously ask what day and hour it was. Sometimes I knew, sometimes I didn't. It was often impossible to figure it out. Even surrounded by people, mine was a world of maddening solitude and darkness.

The nightmare played neatly off of my massive messiah complex. Looking at—and experiencing—the violence done to my body, I had no choice but to deify the pain, to make it holy. I felt the sharp, intrusive needles stabbing me and I felt the metal tubes drilling into my skull and I felt the restraints strangling my hands and arms and I felt the injections on my feet to prevent clotting. Since my pain was so intense, I decided it must be virtuous.

I later understood that technology had saved me. But at the time, it felt as if these were instruments of my destruction.

As I underwent the incessant physical cruelty, my mind provided its own escape. My hallucinations were my only way out.

When the pain grew too intense, Ashok-as-Christ emerged. When I watched my family members—all sitting in chairs, their faces wearing looks of deep agony and despair—I realized I had to save them.

So began my romantic affair with my corporeal self. I would rant daily, "I'm the Body of Love, I'm the Body of Love," as my family looked on in mute, helpless horror. In those moments, I inhaled the world's suffering. All of humanity's dreams, hopes, fantasies, and nightmares lay inside of me, and I never let the doctors and nurses forget it. Whenever they performed their routine tasks, I said solemnly, "Go ahead. My body is ready for you."

My mind whirled through erotic nightmares and dreamscapes as well, involving different genders, fluids, and bleeding and sucking. I recall one hallucination vividly: in my mind, the hospital had a secret orange room, a room of depravity, a room of liberation. It was packed full of women and men of different colors. Some Indian, some Latino, some white, some black. All naked. I remember entering, and running to their bodies like a savage animal and attempting to lick and taste all the flesh they offered.

I remember seeing a gorgeous Indian girl and sucking her nipples till she ripped them off herself out of pain. And when the Latino started exploding in my mouth, his juice wasn't white, but red. It was blood. I was so turned on, and the more aroused I became, the bloodier the room became.

When my eyes opened, I realized there had been no naked bodies, no blood, no oral sex. Just another cruel, surreal mental fiction. That blood I had tasted was liquid food a nurse had been feeding me. I had simply been drinking my meal. The bizarre orgy was just another heightened fantasy to eroticize my internal bleeding, physical anguish, and relentless pain. But my lips felt bloodstained for days.

I was granted three night nurses: Joanna, a tall and haggard white woman; Kiyanna, a sexy young black woman; and Becky, a frumpy redheaded white woman. Becky looked very young, maybe thirty. On one of her nights to watch me—one frightening night—my body changed multiple times.

I broke and then I melted and then I burned.

It started around ten in the evening. Becky had just dimmed my room's lights and closed the door. The first thing I heard was music. Chiming bells, like those from music boxes. Then I looked at my hands. They had become hardened, smooth, and solid white. My light-blue hospital gown had become a light-blue dress. I saw a mirror in front of me. My cheeks were solid white, my lips red, and my eyes glassy and fringed with rigid black eyelashes.

I had become a porcelain doll. Viewing my reflection, I saw my sickening kabuki mask, affixed to my once beautifully brown face. Seeing my newly white cheeks, chin, and nose, I screamed.

My jaws began to tremble. The more I screamed, the more I felt my face being torn apart by the noise. The porcelain doll I had become was breaking, disintegrating. My head, arms, legs, torso, hands, and feet were all breaking into tiny shards. The only thing remaining was the dress.

I screamed again. Without a face, body, or head, the sound emanated from the air itself. After what seemed like an hour, I saw my body materialize again and return to its usual mahogany-colored, fleshy self. Wanting to reassure myself that I was okay, I attempted to touch my face.

But I couldn't; my hands were tied to the bedposts.

I simply shut my eyes and tried to sleep again. Within moments, I felt my body morph to porcelain hardness and then soften back to its normal skin. But then I felt my body soften even further, my flesh becoming looser, limper, thicker and gummier. Though I feared what was happening, I opened my eyes. Again, my body had changed. The skin color was no longer brown, but reddish, the color of wet earth. Terracotta. I had become a doll, again. This time made of clay. But before I could even open my mouth in terror, the clay began changing shape. I was melting, like the Wicked Witch of the West at the end of *The Wizard of Oz.*

Please Lord, let this nightmare end, let me return to normal, I prayed. No such luck. From the melted mire, my figure transformed once more. This time I had become straw. Now I was Raggedy Andy. I suddenly saw small glints of light on my straw feet. Fire. It moved up my feet to my legs to my chest to my arms to my shoulders. It didn't dare touch my head, which, fortunately, had retained its natural form.

In just a few seconds my entire body was in flames, straw burning with unbearable heat. Just as I had never felt the porcelain break, or the clay melt, I never felt the burning of the straw. I thought of chaste Hindu wives who, once upon a time, would immolate themselves after their husbands died.

While my body burned away, I shut my eyes again, only opening them after the sounds of crackling had died.

Gone was the straw. My body had returned.

The porcelain had broken. The clay had melted. The straw had burned. An hour after my shape-shifting hallucination ended, Becky entered the room to check on me. Wearing an unrehearsed smile, she approached my bed.

"I came in because the room was so quiet," she said. "You seemed so peaceful. I bet you must have been having a beautiful dream."

After the depraved sex and terrifying transformations, I

underwent a spectacular religious revelation that would also remain with me forever. I saw death.

No, that's wrong. I saw the afterlife.

Yet rather than seeing the proverbial white light, I entered glorious, deep blue water, and emerged fishlike, making my way through a liquid passage, a magnificent cosmic uterus. I was pushed through a thick wetness to emerge newly born. Dying, it seemed, was as difficult as being born.

The work a newborn endures to leave the womb seemed akin to my struggle; I forced my way through the watery birth canal, to die and be reborn anew.

I discovered the world after death. But just as I was pushing hardest through the heavy fluid, I was stopped—my nurse was slapping my face. It seemed my blood pressure had dropped dangerously low; there was fear for my life. As my death illusion revealed, my hallucinations revealed a new form of consciousness I had never known.

The liquidity taught me that in death we return to being the fish we were in our mothers' wombs. And we enter another, far more substantial womb. Whether this was, indeed, God—as mother, as woman—setting us free once more, or whether the world beyond was a liquid afterlife, I knew that our visions of the hereafter—simple constructs like heaven and hell—meant nothing.

A joy, an exuberance, lay beyond. But it was neither light nor white. It was dark and blue.

Temporal: Spraying Pee and Gagging Free

For the three months preceding the drilling of my skull, a surgical pipe was shoved into the hole of my penis—a catheter to offset my loss of bladder control.

I begged to have the catheter removed. It wasn't. When it finally was, it was the worst pain I'd ever experienced. The nurse laughed. She told me that now I knew what having a baby felt like. She was wrong. Having your dickhole penetrated by a surgical pipe has to feel far worse. Otherwise, surely humankind would have disappeared years ago.

Another horrible intrusion was made through my nose. After a month or so in the hospital, I had stopped eating, and had lost a mighty thirty pounds. The doctors were scared that I would not be strong enough to withstand the open brain surgery, so they inserted a feeding tube.

This nightmarish, pliable tube contained liquid nutrients, which flowed through the nose and directly into the stomach. Another way to feed is to insert the tube directly into the stomach. I wish I had had that one, because then it wouldn't have to pass down my throat.

This method was horrendous. I gagged constantly, hoping to dislodge the plastic from my esophagus. I relentlessly fought the nurses, trying to pull it out.

One time, it all went too far.

It was far past midnight. As usual, I was all alone; I wasn't allowed to have visitors during the night hours.

My nurse that evening was a burly woman named Janet, an intimidating creature whose dark brown hands stood out against my pale hospital gown. I tried to remove the tube. I was choking, coughing, and spitting blood.

"Stop it!" Janet shouted. "I'm warning you, stop it! You're only making it worse for yourself!"

Barely conscious, I kept trying to pull the wicked snake from my nasal passageway, from down inside my throat.

"I warned you!" she screamed.

Suddenly, she pounced, grabbing my arms and pulling them to the sides of my body. She placed a huge hand on my face, preventing me from moving my head at all. Then she punched me hard in the chest.

"You like that? Now you know not to touch the damn tube!"

I was trying to scream, but I couldn't. My face bruised from the force of her grasp. I weighed only one hundred and ten pounds; Janet weighed at least two hundred. The next morning my face and chest were marked black and blue. I screamed to the doctors and my family that Janet had physically abused me. But they considered me delirious; not one person believed me.

Two nights later, Janet was scheduled to be my night nurse again. When I found out, I shrieked and demanded someone else. My wish was finally granted. As for the hellish tube, I pleaded with the doctors to remove it, insisting that my mouth, tongue, and throat had been scraped raw. They told me that it could be removed if I promised to eat food on my own.

From then on, I made sure to keep my mouth full of food whenever the doctors passed. Even the hospital Jell-O couldn't be as bad as the alternative.

Arachnoid: The Last Supper

My craniotomy was scheduled for May 5, barely one week after my nurse had beaten me up.

On the evening before, I was supposed to be relaxed and peaceful, since I would be facing the most grueling experience of my life. I had been in great spirits all day, laughing and joking with the doctors. *What the hell,* they must have been thinking, *let's make him laugh!*

One more head shave was necessary, and the man to do it was Dr. Khan. An Egyptian transplant, he always reassured me with a warm smile and kind words. As he shaved my head, he decided to try his hand at comedy.

"Hey Ashok," he said as the razor grazed my head, "you ever think about being a singer?"

"What's that question all about?"

"I was just thinking that with the turban you're going to wear, you could be a backup singer for Erykah Badu."

"Lame," I responded, but I was silently pleased that he was even attempting to use Erykah Badu as a comic prop.

Dad had promised to bring me dinner from TGI Friday's.

Meals from outside were usually against regulations, but he was given special permission, since my head would be carved the next day. I requested chicken fingers and French fries.

At 7:30, Mom, Dad, Prakash, Karmen, and I were sitting in my hospital room, telling stories. The TGI Friday's meal had just been placed on my lap. Damn, it looked good.

Just then my personal terror walked in. It was Janet. On this night, before the big operation, she was my nurse.

"Get her out!" I shrieked. "She tried to murder me! Get that demon out!"

I continued screaming as Janet moved closer, causing my blood pressure to shoot up.

Before, few had believed my story about Janet abusing me. However, Prakash trusted me. At no time during my entire stay had I claimed I had been thrashed by anyone else.

Prakash quickly called one of the doctors working on the floor. Dr. Williams had never dealt with me, but she knew about my case. A white woman of about sixty, with inappropriate waist-length gray hair, she seemed exhausted when Prakash spoke to her.

"Tomorrow's Ashok's craniotomy, Dr. Williams. But there's one issue we haven't dealt with?" he said.

"Which one? He just has to stay calm," Dr. Williams responded.

"Right. But Janet's his night nurse again; she mauled him before and now he's freaking out."

"Impossible. She has an impeccable record. She wouldn't do that."

Prakash remained calm. "I'm not going to argue with you about that now, doctor. All we know is that he is not in good shape, and needs to rest."

Dr. Williams finally agreed. "Okay, here's what I'll do. I'll send over Dr. Babu to give him a sedative. And I'll call the head nurse to tell her about this."

Prakash returned to the bed and recounted what Dr. Williams said. Dr. Babu was a fat, jovial Indian man. Originally from New Delhi, he had come to America just a year prior. He was charming and relaxed, and Tribe Rajamani dug him.

The head nurse was Priscilla, a wonderfully kind woman. She was black, very short, very muscular, very dark, very beautiful. She had amazing bedside manners. She decided that she would take care of me that night.

My family was relieved.

Dr. Babu came in and gave me a powerful sedative. I didn't know what that drug was, but oh my God, everyone should try it. It not only calmed me down, it made me feel as if I were on a sandy beach in the Bahamas.

Janet began to leave the room. Prakash suddenly cornered her.

"What exactly happened that night?"

"I don't know, I was just doing my job," she said, looking away and speaking like a little child.

"Ashok is adamant in claiming that you hurt him."

"I'm sorry if he was bothered, Mr. Rajamani," she continued in her little girl voice. "I might have been a little forceful. Sometimes nurses have no other option."

"But he was so feeble! Plus he didn't know what he was doing at all."

"Once again, I'm sorry." She rushed out.

I was relocated to a new room, under the care of Priscilla. Everything was right with the world. But there was a downside to the victory. My TGI Friday's chicken fingers and fries had grown cold. I was forced to eat the evening specialty from the hospital cafeteria: chewy steak and canned peas. And the Holy Grail for the Last Supper? Not a pre–*Da Vinci Code* chalice of ornately decorated glass, but a large plastic mug of vanilla protein drink. Shortly after I ate my feast, the lovely pills submerged me into a guiltless sleep.

Soon, very soon, my skull would be drilled wide open.

Not the First Time in Jail:
1989–1992

Yes, I'm a Dirty Dothead!

The pain inflicted on me in the hospital wasn't completely surprising. I had been Abu-Ghraib'd before.

Grayslake Community High School was the first jail in which I had been imprisoned. I was thirteen when my sentence began, and as I entered GCHS for freshman year, panic struck me. I was puny when I first saw the dingy three-story building, just a few inches over five feet, and still wearing thick spectacles. My bushy black hair had grown past my chin, too straight to be considered an Indo-fro, but poufy and thick and dry enough to resemble brittle, licorice-flavored cotton candy. The summer sun had darkened my skin, and the only meat on my bony figure protruded from my stomach, causing a substantially distended gut.

I could easily have been the poster child for a Sally Struthers "Save the Children" Fund.

Wearing a blue Ocean Pacific tee and Lee corduroys that I had purchased specifically for the first day of school, I felt handsome, although the outfit only accentuated my emaciation.

Once the sterile metal doors banged shut behind me, I had officially been incarcerated in a world that would make me long for the glory days of Ass-Hock and show-and-tell face-offs. This inferno was as obscenely white as Avon, but since it was filled with worldly teens instead of innocent kids, I was greeted with a barrage of sophisticated racism from the very first day.

The summer before, I made the mistake of watching *Grease* and *Grease 2* marathons on TV. Each movie depicted high-schoolers who looked old and used enough to be chain-smoking empty nesters. I discussed the problem with Prakash, who had already inhabited this academic universe for a whole three years before me.

"Prakash, is it true that all the kids in high school look so old?"

"Even older."

"What are you talking about? That Rizzo looks like she could be someone's grandma!"

"Sorry, Ashok, the kids look even older than Rizzo."

I was surprised to find out that he wasn't exactly joking. The other students were freakishly tall and massive, featuring stubbled boys and beyond busty girls. I couldn't believe these kids were only thirteen. *Oh well,* I thought, *let them greet this kid who looks like a malnourished Ethiopian midget.*

For me, freshman life was a never-ending blur of slurs and name-calling. I was getting good grades, but nothing could compensate for the terrors that took place.

In addition to occasionally speaking to me with an exaggerated Indian accent, many of my classmates, especially the "popular" or "jock" stars, flung me a lovely collection of monikers that first year, such as "Sandman" (Indians, they figured, were like Arabs, and hence came from deserts); "Camel Jockey" (same premise); "Dirty Gandhi" (self-explanatory); and "Dothead" (self-explanatory, squared).

After one sweaty hour of knee football, which was like regular football except that we played it on our knees (sounds sexier than it was), I received a lovely keepsake in the locker room. Two of the jocks forcibly wrapped a wet towel on my head, saying that it's what my family wore anyway.

Prakash didn't save me when we both shared time in the hellhole. I wondered why. I also wondered when at home he never spoke about the racism at school. I figured that perhaps because I was a lot smaller than his large frame, I was the only one attacked.

One Friday, though, I witnessed tall, muscular Prakash opening his locker to find a magazine photo of a nameless turbaned Sikh covered with red crosses and the phrase, "Go Home."

So that's why he never spoke about high school, I realized. *He's getting as much shit as me.* The only difference was that he kept it to himself.

The attacks continued the next year, although there were a few new additions. For example, the slave joke: If someone asked for a favor, like picking up a fallen pencil, the responder wouldn't do it, instead replying, "What color does my skin look like? Ashok's?"

Bush One's Persian Gulf War provided new fodder for the white teen masses hungry for South Asian blood.

Sauntering to my chemistry class, I heard some of the jock boys speaking loudly in the gray-tiled hallway. Not paying close attention, instead thinking about the test I hadn't studied for, I figured they were just high-fiving each other over some random ball game. Then I tripped. Burly blond Todd had stuck his leg in front of my right foot. When I stood up again, he spoke to me as loudly as possible.

"Ashok, guess what? We found a new name for you: 'Fucking Iraqi.'"

There must have been laughter, but I didn't give a damn at that moment. I was still concerned about memorizing the periodic table.

But from that day on, I started paying attention. I was, indeed, now dubbed "Fucking Iraqi."

"Go back to Iraq and quit killing our soldiers" was a common phrase directed to me.

One day after gym class, I couldn't take it any longer. Terrence, a tiny white boy with a sandy-brown bowl cut, had been barking the Iraqi nickname. I finally let loose and punched his stomach. Suddenly, we two scrawny midget boys were fighting. Before we knew it, a substantial crowd of more than ten classmates had gathered. They sang. A sweet, brief, one verse sing-a-long:

"A fight! A fight! Sand nigger and a white!"

Unfortunately, before the melody could become an anthemic pop wonder, grouchy old Mrs. Baumgard from the nearby biology classroom came storming down the hallway. By the time she reached us, all of the kids had cleverly dispersed, and she found Terrence and me on the floor. After separating us and shooing him back to class, she spoke to me. Only to me.

"Never provoke a fight again, Ashok," she said.

I would obey.

Lady of the House

In the second semester of sophomore year, we had an assignment in history class to write about a pivotal moment in America. I wrote about World War II and the Japanese-American internment camps. As I researched this era, I had a weird reaction: I was jealous. At least *they were with their own kind*.

As bad as school was becoming, there was good news on the home front: finally, another family of color was moving into Quail Creek. The newcomers were a black family called the Taylors. One mom, one dad, and one lovely teenage daughter, Karen. Mom happily brought over her special welcome wagon of coconut rice. After just three weeks of settling in, they told Mom they had to take a quick trip to Atlanta, for a family emergency. Upon their return to our community, they noticed blue graffiti sprayed on their townhouse.

GET OUT NIGGERS.

They moved out of Grayslake immediately. Seems they followed orders perfectly.

Throughout everything, I begged Dad to move. He refused; after all, his work was in Chicago, and we could afford the mortgage for our Quail Creek townhouse.

One afternoon while I was doing my homework, the doorbell rang. Mom went to the door, worried about finding a Jehovah's Witness, but was instead confronted by a tall, white, middle-aged dish network salesman.

I overhead their brief conversation.

In minimal makeup and barely-there lipstick, she was dressed in a simple white tee and gray flat-front trousers, and looked effortlessly glamorous.

"Hi!" she said, smiling at the man.

"Hello, may I speak to your boss please?"

"Pardon me?" she said, confused.

The salesman sighed, as if he were doing a favor by deigning to talk to her again.

"I said, may I speak to the Lady of the House, please?"

"That's me," she responded with a sigh.

We knew, once again, that nothing had changed. Mom could be a fairy-tale queen, wearing regal red robes and a glittering crown as she glided through a glittering ballroom, in a moated castle of precious marble and stone. If this castle was in America, she would still be asked if she was the maid.

Sweet Dreams

As I had enjoyed creating art ever since I was three, drawing and painting images both figurative and abstract, I took multiple fine arts classes. In Figure Painting I, I met a beautiful girl named Kayla Moore. She was a contrast from all the other Teutonic students in the school: her father was white, her mother black. She had full, gorgeous lips, which of course were labeled by the students as "nigger lips," Angelina Jolie and collagen having yet to make their marks on our culture. Kayla was curvy and petite, shorter than me, with long, waist-length bronze curls that highlighted her dark golden skin. I was infatuated with her, but was too afraid to ask her out on a date. Being such an outsider had subconsciously affected my sense of teen conventionality, so I simply didn't have romances.

In the same class, I made friends with Joel Tomasetti, who, like Kayla, was different from the masses. His parents were from Sicily. With olive skin and an ebony crew cut, he was wonderfully eccentric, insisting on painting fake plastic fruit in most of his canvases. His height matched mine, yet because he was a gym-bot, he was conspicuously muscular, not merely toned.

Ever since seventh grade, when I first heard about "cumming," I had been jerking off on a weekly basis, hoping I would finally release what the kids called "jizz." It never worked. The "J" word was still foreign to my body.

Finally it happened, very, very late, at the age of fifteen.

I was asleep at the time, waking up to a sticky mess on my stomach. *My first wet dream,* I thought.

But then I realized what I had been dreaming about.

Kayla had been fucking me.

So, too, had Joel.

The Motherland and the Great Escape

Even though my life in Grayslake continued being a nightmare, I had been granted parole on occasion, one month each. My parents had taken Prakash and me to Mumbai on five summer odysseys. I would relish everything about the city: the tastes, the smells, the sights—from the moment our planes arrived at Sahar Airport, now renamed Chatrapati Shivaji International Airport in honor of seventeenth-century Emperor Chatrapati Shivaji Raje Bhonsle. Great leader, yes. Catchy airport name, hell no.

Like any major international destination, the airport was not located in the city center—just as JFK and LaGuardia were not located in Times Square—but was located in the surrounding neighborhood of Andheri. As soon as we entered the airport, I knew a missing piece of my heart had been replaced, momentarily, at least the part that needed drama, energy, and sweet suffocation. We would always arrive in India at the ungodly hour of 4 a.m. Never changed. No flight, it appeared, could ever reach this enormous city in the midst of daylight, or in the traditional scape of nighttime. After trying to navigate through the storm of travelers to the visitors' passport line, we would pick up our luggage before heading to customs. Since our family was of Indian blood, the airport officials spoke only Marathi to us. Luckily, this was the language of Mom's childhood, so after she joked and giggled, and occasionally flirted with the security guys, we passed through quickly and easily.

Once we finally left the terminal doors, it dawned on me: *this was India.* The first thing that hit was the heat, an immense heat that overwhelmed me with its gorgeous unbearability. Next came the smell. This was not the odor of cabbies or the restaurants in Manhattan's Little India. Scents mingled in the steamy air, assaulting me like a punch in the face, the smell of double-decker buses that squeezed between motionless cars, and of cows that nonchalantly strolled the streets. No, this was not about sweaty, unwashed men; this was the smell of a universe in which humankind coexisted with animals, coexisted with congested heat, and coexisted with fragrances that surprised as well as amazed.

It was natural that with so many people, the air was ripe

with stress, though not the emotional kind, but the type in which people were late to work and had to hurry, babies' cries were drowned by rickshaws stalling, and pedestrians were so frustrated they were yelling at the air above, not at the streets below.

India was a world of contrasts. Orthodox priests, in saffron robes and holy threads, were driving mopeds. Farm animals stopped at crosswalks. This was God's backyard: a family reunion with a messy barbeque, and pets running throughout, and neighbors sunbathing.

Perhaps the most wondrous thing for me was the ocean of beautiful brown skin around me. After all, I was a brown-skinned boy in a small Bible Belt town in the heart of all-white America. I never felt attractive, or even human for that matter.

In India, I could finally discover this beauty of recognition in others, and it was amazing. When I would look up, down, left, right, I would see people that looked liked me. Same eyes, noses, mouths, pigments. I was alive at last, a human being with a beauty seen throughout the streets. Each person I saw was a reflection in a mirror I desperately needed. Perhaps this was why I had such a viscerally angry reaction to the white faces peeking through — the European backpackers, the rich white American women on their quest for spiritual healing via Oprah's book club. I was finally, after all, entering a land smothered in colors I could never experience in my daily life.

The joke, however, was that, deep in the pit of my redneck soul, I didn't believe I was even considered Indian when I went to the subcontinent. Just a "damn dirty Yank," to paraphrase Charleton Heston's infamous words of contempt leveled at the apes in the movie *The Planet of the Apes*.

While these trips to India typically included my family, I finally traveled there alone, the summer before my junior year at GCHS. The experience was life-changing. Rather than head to Mumbai, this time I chose to travel to multiple cities, including New Delhi, Agra, Jaipur, and Kerala, uncovering religious centers of the many diverse Indian faiths. I saw the famed Snake temple, Taj Mahal, Jami Masjid mosque, and the Sikh Golden Temple. I even made a pilgrimage to Gandhi's tomb, walking down the path where the Mahatma himself walked as he was assassinated.

We Have Overcome

Newly empowered, I returned to high school a different person. My hair, parted down the middle, had grown very long, falling past my shoulders, and I now wore circle-framed spectacles instead of my trademark squares.

I had become John Lennon with a tan. Additionally, I had bulked up, my body having packed on a mighty twenty more pounds, and I had grown to what would be my final adult height. A new Ashok reentered GCHS that fall. No longer fearing my white, popular peers, I started attaching myself, with a vengeance, to different cliques, like the goths, alterna-punks, skaters, art elites, stoners, and, of course, nerds.

We now assembled a Warholian factory, a demimonde of outcasts, underdogs, and subversives. In addition to my buds Kayla and Joel, there was Tom, the geekish loner who read Stephen Hawking; Steven, who worshiped Satan; Chris, the boy who wore mascara and red lipstick; Karla, who could barely stand, pumped full of narcotics. And of course, all six students of color in the entire school: Missy, Lila, and Doug, the token black kids; Sam the Korean; Emilio the Mexican. And me.

On graduation day, after finally surviving our nightmarish high school years, "the Factory" sashayed through the halls, shouting "We Have Overcome."

Most of the kids in my town weren't headed for college. After graduation, many were arrested for minor felonies, or had babies who would likely end up playing with the pink flamingos that vamped in their yards. SATs were never discussed in GCHS, and my guidance counselor guided me toward a local junior-vocational institute. I eventually took the tests on my own, however, and actually applied to a few four-year universities, vowing never, ever to return to Illinois.

I chose to attend New York University.

But what else could a Baby Buddha do?

Wasn't the Big Apple the only possible destination for a fleeing Midwesterner?

The Incarceration, Part Two:
2000 (IV)

Dura: Cinco De Mayo

On May 5, 2000, my skull was opened.

An unseen nurse wheeled me into the operating room. It's strange, but I swear it was my linebacker-abuser Janet. Or was it Satan, Mephistopheles himself? Let's just call her Janestopheles. She could have been the one who rolled me in. Perhaps in that moment, my subconscious mind was thinking of a possible postsurgery death, via a non-Hindu highway. Perhaps I had envisioned not a Kingdom of Heaven but a Kingdom of Hell.

Here now, a gripping recap of the subsequent thirteen-hour operation, none of which I remember of course:

1. At 7 a.m. anesthesia was shot into my arm, rendering me unconscious. I was placed facedown on a rotating operating table, my arms spread wide, my head tightly secured in

a viselike contraption. The visual effect was that of being nailed to an upside-down crucifix, which was perfect for my Messiah complex.

2. After incisions were traced across it, my naked skull was penetrated by an instrument cruelly and inaccurately called the "Midas Rex" drill, as if this procedure was going to transform my brain into gold.

3. My skull plate was then lifted away and placed into a sterile salt solution, so it would be shiny and new when it was screwed back in. My brain was now naked to the air.

4. The surgeons started cutting into the messy goo. The leftover AVM was coagulated with a form of glue into an electrified removable ball, then taken out completely. Blood was drained, the brain was fully cleaned and irrigated, and four metal clips were stapled inside to discipline the remaining veins. No more tangles.

5. Drumroll please—my skull was brought back from its salt-bath and returned to its proper position. Four titanium plates were placed over the entire puzzle, and steel screws secured them onto the bone.

6. The reattached piece of skull, now outlined with heavy metal, was in the shape of a horseshoe.

Cortex: Family-in-Waiting

An account of the seemingly never-ending surgery would not be complete, of course, unless accompanied by the seemingly never-ending wait. As my head was opened and closed, my family held their vigil. Mom, Dad, Prakash, and Karmen began their marathon sofa-warming in the waiting room at 5 a.m. and had carved near-perfect buttock grooves into the furniture cushions by the time the butchery ended at 8 p.m.

The room had peach carpeting, white walls, and in the middle, a large grouping of bamboo planted firmly in a red glass vase. A television screen was secured on a wall.

The four Rajamanis claimed two of the plush blue sofas in the surprisingly crowded room. Twelve other people were there, also waiting for their loved ones.

As the amount of time increased, so did my family's fears and anxieties. Mom began cataloging and then endlessly reviewing the list of possible consequences: total blindness, total deafness, total paralysis.

Prakash finally verbalized what everyone had been thinking: "He could die."

Mom looked away.

The wait was toughest for Dad, a recovering heart patient himself. He couldn't handle stress very well, and this stress was overwhelming. As he stood up to stretch, his eyes closed.

"What's wrong with you?" Mom asked.

Dad's body began to sway. He quickly reached out to grab an arm of the sofa, but pawed the air instead. Then he collapsed on the carpet. Karmen and Mom screamed. Nurses rushed in. Their prescription? A cup of orange juice. Strange, but it did the trick. Dad slowly gained complete consciousness.

Karmen brought him sugar cookies from the cafeteria and then she walked him up and down the hallway. Dad stopped to look at a large aquarium. The fish calmed him. Dad didn't collapse again.

When the surgery was over, two of the surgeons informed my family that I was fine, but explained that I was extremely fragile, and nobody could visit me for a while.

But they also had come to know my family during my long stay here, so they permitted one person to see me in the postsurgery area. Dad had just collapsed and Mom would be a wreck if she saw my head looking like a horse-hide baseball. Everybody decided that Prakash was the guy to do it.

He climbed into a standard blue hospital gown and put on a surgical mask and gloves. When he entered the room, he was horrified.

I was wrapped, head to toe, in bandages. There were five or six plastic tubes jutting out of my skull. My shaved, ravaged head still bore bloodstains, and a clear plastic mask protected my face. Metallic bracelets attached both arms to the bed.

Prakash gaped at me silently for a minute, and then he slowly returned to the lounge.

He described my appearance and told everybody that all the medical attachments made me look like an astronaut

ready to blast off into orbit. He had hoped to put a smile on
my parents' faces.

He failed.

Thalamus: Damage, Divinity

"He's fallen! Oh my God, he's fallen!"

Joanna and Kiyanna shrieked in one piercing voice that
cut through the stillness of the ward. As Becky had permanently left the hospital for another job, these were the only
two protectors paid to take care of me at night.

Forty-eight hours after my open brain surgery, I fell. It
was about 2 a.m. I was in my private room in the hospital's
critical care section.

Back then, I didn't know where I was. But I knew I had to
take a leak. There was a bathroom in the room, so I headed
for it. Sure, there were tubes sticking out of me. But when
nature calls, such details hardly matter.

The next thing I remember, my back was splayed across
the cold tiles and I lay in a jumble of tubes. That's when the
screaming started.

Until that moment, my mind had convinced me that I was
home, safe and sound. My delirium had allowed me to forget
about my time in the hospital, about the bleed, and most of
all, about the surgery. Until that moment, my sole quest was
to reach the bathroom.

When I heard the nursely shrieks, I knew I had done

something wrong. The PICC-line had popped out—a twelve-foot drainage tube needled into my arm and extending to my aorta. I had also dislodged my ventrics, those antlerlike tubes drilled into the bone of my skull. The fall had ripped them all out.

Unaware of the severity of the situation, I laughed with embarrassment. I was just a silly old man who fell while going to the bathroom. "God," I murmured, "I slipped. I'm so retarded."

Kiyanna quickly called my family. I was placed back on the bed, my medical equipment next to my pillow. The doctors were summoned and I was brought to the Intensive Care Unit.

Upon arriving, Mom was too stunned to speak. But Prakash was not at a loss for words:

"WHAT THE HELL IS WRONG WITH YOU TWO," he shouted at the nurses. "YOU BETTER PRAY THAT NOTHING HAS HAPPENED TO HIM!"

Joanna and Kiyanna were not fired, just reprimanded. But everyone felt this incident would prove prophetic. How could I survive, when every single thing that was keeping me alive had been violently ripped from my body?

The next forty-eight hours proved to be the scariest yet. Unfortunately, I was coherent at this point.

I had an emergency MRI and emergency EEG. There was no new damage, but the pain was severe and relentless.

"I'm dying! I'm dying!" I had never screamed so loud. I had never known such agony. I cried for my mother. Only later did I learn she had been by my side all along.

After the MRI, I was whisked to an operating room where the emergency surgeons quickly drilled new ventrics into my head, inserted a new PICC line, and replaced the feeding tubes. The renewed pain was overwhelming. But I was alive.

A few days later, I found myself in Brooklyn, New York. My head was resting in the lap of Lord Krishna in a temple. I was at his altar, deep in the dark inner sanctum, fragrant jasmine flowers and elaborate golden lamps surrounding my limp body. Using an ivory cloth, the Lord was tenderly wiping away the blood cascading from the cracks in my skull, cleansing and purifying my wounded head. I cried in ecstasy as I looked into his eyes.

Returning to the hospital after what seemed like days, I awakened in bed to the warm faces of Mom and Gina, a new nurse hired to take care of me, just a week earlier. She was young, Chinese, and obese.

I shouted to both, "Krishna cleaned me! I was in Brooklyn! I was in a Krishna temple in Brooklyn!"

"Ashok, honey," Gina said gently, "Brooklyn is far away. You are in D.C. Washington D.C. But you've been asleep all day."

"No," I argued, "I was there, and Krishna held me!"

Mom smiled.

"You were just dreaming."

I was not, I knew. I touched my head to check if Krishna had cleansed it thoroughly. He had.

After the Fall, the hospital took no chances. I was permanently restrained in my hospital bed, hands and feet bound. I would now have to stay in the hospital another month, instead of the two weeks initially prescribed.

Hippocampus: Get Up, Stand Tall

I was tied to the bed; all my rights to mobility had been revoked. I couldn't even sit on a chair. But I had one permanent visitor: Mom. She sat in a blue plastic chair, just two feet from my face. She watched silently as I shrieked, responding to my imagined torture sequences. She was unable to do what a mother should: console me. All she could do was sit and stare. But no matter how long or loud I wailed, in my endless delirium, Mom sat in that plastic chair—watching over me helplessly as inner demons plagued me.

One day, a nurse told Mom she had to leave the room. There was probably some needling, blood pumping, or fluid draining to be done. Mom began shouting, refusing to leave her baby's side. One should never mess with a South Indian mother. She created such an uproar that two doctors had to be called in. Only then did she comply. But as soon as she could, Mom returned to the blue plastic chair.

One day I was informed that I would have to leave my bed. My destination was a plush brown La-Z-Boyish chair two feet away. My reaction was a distorted version of the Stockholm Syndrome: I had grown attached to the bed, which, at first, had imprisoned me and tortured me. Now it was my sanctuary, my one place for survival, for security. I didn't want to leave it.

The entire relocation process took less than five minutes. A swift lift of one leg, a turn of an arm, a pull of a shoulder, and I was finally sitting upright.

It was an unfamiliar and unwanted experience at first, but I quickly learned to love it. I was surprised how great it felt to be sitting upright.

For the next week, I ruled from my brown throne. But there was yet another transition to make, from the plush cushion to a metal seat. This one had wheels.

My very own wheelchair, I thought lovingly. I had been placed in my mobile home. I could move at last.

For the first time in nearly three months, I was free. That is, free enough to keep a smile on my face, my dimples emerging once more. Wheeled from corridor to corridor, I grinned happily, waving to everyone.

I was Miss America. No, I was a Queen. Cleopatra, Elizabeth, you name it. I was a maharani from Rajput palaces.

My newfound pleasure, however, was quickly crushed when I learned of my next challenge: I would have to walk.

On my own two legs. It was too soon, I thought, I had just started to enjoy my gray chariot. How the fuck could I walk, logistically speaking? I was attached to a huge IV pole. Sure, it kept me alive, but it was a bulky instrument that I had grown to loathe.

I begged not to have to do it. But even timid nurses can exert their power. A scrawny Filipino nurse named Chan became my disciplinarian.

"If you don't walk now, you will *never* be able to walk again," he threatened.

"I'm not ready for this," I whined.

"Do you want to be handicapped? Crippled in a wheelchair? If that's what you want, then stay in your wheelchair."

"Fuck you."

"Use your legs, pussy."

That did it. *I'll show him*, I thought. True, I may have been less than 120 pounds, and I may not have seen my manhood for months, but I sure was no pussy. Queen, maybe. Pussy, no.

It was time for the baby to walk.

I was lifted out of the wheelchair, my lumbering IV pole still attached to me. For what felt like the first time in my life, my frail feet met the cold white tiles. Kiyanna helped me stand straight, hold tightly to the pole and begin walking. Immediately, Mom joined Chan, and both held one side of my body, as I clung fiercely to my pole.

Never had I felt so terrified.

I was maneuvered to the long hallway. At the other end was Kiyanna, who had quickly scampered to be there. My mission was to reach her. Fifteen feet looked like fifty yards.

At that moment, I remembered being a toddler years ago in New Jersey, running for the first time into Mommy's arms. I had been a late bloomer, learning to walk when I was a two-year-old. Now at the age of twenty-five, I was a late bloomer all over again.

Medulla: The Mom Diaries

Sitting in the garish blue plastic chair next to the hospital bed, Mom could do nothing to save her son as he groaned and screamed and fought against restraints. So she wrote letters.

March 23, 2000
Dear God,

It has been less than a week since Ashok's in the hospital. Nothing makes sense to me. We had all come to share in the joy and happiness of Prakash and Karmen on their wedding day, and Ashok is in the ICU fighting for his life. Why did it all have to happen at this time? Ashok has just started his new job, a responsible position, and off to a great start. I hope I'm providing him some solace and comfort, and I hope he knows I'm there in the room.

March 26, 2000
My dear Ashok,

Your condition is bad. Fever is way up. It's been 8 days since you were admitted. Some days I wonder what is my reality and yours as I sit by your bedside in the ICU. There is a world moving outside, getting on with their daily chores. Mine has come to a standstill. There is no escape or exit for both of us. Maybe in a few weeks we will see that exit.

I'm sitting in the ICU waiting room, and I strike up a conversation with another mom. Her 32-years-old son has had a hemorrhage. She's a priestess of a church in D.C. She comes and sits next to me, holds my hand, praises the name of Lord Jesus, and asks me to put my hands together, blesses me and tells me that the healing hands of a mother is the only way to bring a child back to life, and that this moment shall pass and that my child will be okay. Healing words and two mothers in pain sharing a moment. For just that moment there was a calm, as loneliness and solitude go hand in hand in the waiting rooms of all hospitals.

March 28, 2000
Dear God,

Watch over Ashok, let him be well and come back to us, the pep in his spoken words and his thinking intact. His brain has been hurt. It's 3 p.m. I am teary-eyed as I watch Ashok restrained and lying so helplessly in the bed.

Keep Ashok in good spirit dear God, despite his pain, and relieve him of some of his pain. His eyes are glazed and time is standing still.

March 29, 2000
My dear Ashok,

Another afternoon, some laughter heard. There is this anti-septic feeling, where all lives hang in the balance, and for each of us it is this slow process of looking for that little light at the end of the road, where there might be slight improve-ment, and the day we could finally take our loved ones home. Ashok, you are so disoriented today.

I feel so helpless.

April 2, 2000
Dear God,

Please spare his eyes. He's an artist. Spare his eyes. I know God, I'm asking a lot from you.

April 17, 2000
My dear Prakash and Karmen,

Thank you for your birthday wishes, and thank you for the couple of hours at the hair stylist for a cut. For those few hours I felt a little sense of normalcy. Before long I hope Ashok will get a chance to get a haircut and shave and come back to us.

May 4, 2000
My dear Ashok,

I sense calmness and a bit of nervousness with the impending surgery. I am so glad that you are conscious and will ask the Dr. all the right questions. You signed the waiver too, quite in control. In two days you will be fighting the biggest battle of your life in the OR, Ashok. Know that I love you dearly and want you to fight hard and come back to us alive and kicking. Know that Dad, Prakash, Karmen and I are sending you all our positive energies.

June 20, 2000
Dear Ashok,

This is your biggest test now that you fought hard to come back to us. There is so much you have to do in this life. Think pleasant thoughts as the nightmare is over. Laughter, smiles, fluffy clouds, blue waters and sunny skies await you.

Love always, Mom

Formatting Ashok Version 2.0: 2000 (V)

Sunshiny Day

I was finally freed in the first week of July.

My first experience in the outside world was a revelation. Newborns usually cry at birth, although not because of pain. Babies squeal because they are physiologically adapting to a jolting new world outside of the womb. It is the first time they exit their warm, wet homes and confront cold, dry space. It is the first time their lungs breathe air. And it is the first time they are exposed to light.

Until now, I had been lodged in another womb. The NCCU, the Neuro-critical Care Unit, was the remote domain of victims of stroke, bleeds, hemorrhages, and all traumatic brain injuries. This dark, confined world was the hospital's hushed, isolated realm for neurological patients.

The craniotomy whisked away some of that darkness. I was slowly working up toward feeling that full light on my face.

One week before I was released, I had to visit a neuro-ophthalmologist. He was located in another building on the hospital campus. This was a major event; it would be the first time I was outside after the seeming eternity of three bed-ridden months.

Even though I had relearned how to walk—at least rudimentarily and awkwardly, like a blind supermodel walking down an oil-slicked catwalk—I was placed in a wheelchair for my first trip outdoors.

A superanimated young man named Nate wheeled me to the building. He was a welcome change from the typically somber hospital staff. My mother walked beside him. Whereas I was in my rumpled hospital gown, he was in a fresh uniform. It was solid white, in stunning contrast to his ebony skin. His huge body maneuvered my small, weakened frame along the sidewalk.

Until now, I had been languishing in the dark, blinded. But when Nate wheeled me out of my prison, everything changed within a second. He had become my angel on earth, my divine healer.

I felt air—genuine, outside air—flowing into my body. I felt the clouds and blue sky hug me. I saw the sun and felt its heat. I had just been released from the black sphere within my head into the world, a world of brightness, a world of freedom, and a world of light. The sun symbolized everything that was active and breathing. And I was finally aglow with it. I had truly re-entered the land of the living.

"Look, there's the sun!" I yelled to Mom and Nate.

In Hinduism, the oldest scripture, the Vedas, glorifies the sun as a vital deity named Surya. In fact, the brahmanical rite—the thread ceremony—involves placing a holy thread on a young man with a hymn to the sun, to divine illumination. This ceremony is the Hindu equivalent of a bar mitzvah. Part of the ritual is a prayer in which the youth interlocks his hands, placing them directly on his face, then looks at the sun and prays.

I had previously experienced the ritual myself. But at that time, I found it difficult to believe in its importance. When I was younger, I scoffed at some of the superstitions in ancient Hinduism. Like most religions, its early form involved the deification of elements: the sun, moon, fire, air, water, and earth. I once considered it naïve to worship this way.

But after my "sun experience," I had, to some degree, a change of mind. Why are most children and adults intrigued by fire? Why do the sun and moon hold a grip on our imaginations? We know the science behind all these entities, but still, they hold a magical influence over us.

Certainly, I was affected by what I witnessed that day. I had, in a way, realized a higher power. Perhaps the ancient gurus, with all their silly fears and superstitions, were right after all. Perhaps the elements indeed possess divinity.

My sight would never be the same again. But I had new eyes, and a new way of seeing.

The Hotel

The doctors insisted my family and I stay for a while in a nearby Washington hotel, before going to my parents' home in New Jersey. We couldn't risk another medical mishap like my fall. This time, I was given another metal companion: a massive IV pole that continuously delivered powerful antibiotics.

I hated my new posse member. I couldn't walk anywhere without lugging him around. Moving with him seemed to be an exercise in animism: When I looked at him, I swear I could see his mocking smile.

My parents administered daily injections of essential post-surgical intravenous antibiotics. Our insurance didn't cover daily personal nurses after hospitalization, so my parents became my caregivers. They had to dose me every three hours, through my arm's PICC line, which jutted from the inside of my elbow.

"Homecare" nurses came every few days to make sure my parents performed these duties correctly. I had little confidence in my parents' work, especially when they made my skin bleed.

During that time, we had an interesting guest, one of the few relatives we have in this country. My father's brother came to visit from Texas. A wiry, wheat-skinned Indian man, Ramanan Uncle was a welcome addition to our second-rate hospice. He had oversized spectacles and a bushy, almost cartoonish mustache. A hard-working pharmacist, he carefully guided my parents in their work. He made me feel less bitter about the IV pole, inviting me to mail it to him after I was free from it. Most important, his presence curbed my parents' frequent arguments. At the time, he meant everything to me. I adored him.

Away from the hospital, everyday rituals now became a source of embarrassment. Bathing was the worst. I had to be washed by my mother. I know it was no big issue to her, but I just couldn't deal with it. I could accept my nurses bathing me, but this was different.

Luckily, I was often drugged out at bathtime, which spared me some mortification at being soaped up like a baby in the tub. After rinsing my body, Mom would shampoo my hair, or what had grown back so far; this was the only positive aspect of the entire ordeal. Since I had received only sponge baths in the hospital, I had forgotten the wonderful sensation of free-flowing water. Mom gently lathered my hair and poured water on it from a small jug. It felt as if God herself was pouring divine nectar on my bruised skull. Those moments of joy were rare. I typically felt an overwhelming sadness. I was sad to be unable to function as a "normal" adult, sad to be unable to perform a simple activity I had once taken for granted, and sad to be a baby, once again bathed by *Mommy*.

Homeless (or, Life in Cardboard)

The morning before we left the hotel to travel to my parents' home in New Jersey, Mom confessed something that nearly induced another hemorrhage. While Dad and Ramanan Uncle were sleeping in their respective bedrooms, not yet arisen at 8 a.m., she cornered me in the blue-tiled kitchenette of the large hotel suite.

Thirsty for water, I was reaching for a glass, when she tapped my shoulder, surprising me.

"Ashok," she said tenderly, "let me make you some tea."

"Thanks," I muttered groggily.

"By the way, I have to confess something. Go sit down, and I'll bring the tea."

She looked worried as she carried in the two cups. I was already seated on one end of the uncomfortable wicker couches in the living room. She sat next to me. She had made tasty tea. It was chamomile, with a dab of honey.

"While you were hospitalized," she began apprehensively, "Your father . . ."

"Yes?"

"He broke your apartment lease."

I thought she was joking, and I began chuckling.

"He broke the lease, removed every single belonging from your studio apartment."

"You're just playing with me, right? Dad wouldn't do that."

"I wish it weren't true. I tried to tell him not to, but he was so adamant."

She rubbed her eyes.

"So where's my stuff?" I asked, suddenly angry.

"He packed everything in cardboard cartons and placed them in our garage."

Seeing my face, which was turning stormier as she continued speaking, she said, "Ashok, he didn't know what he was doing, he didn't know what would happen to you! You have to forgive him!"

I nodded, but I didn't know what hurt more: the idea that I was now homeless, or the fact that by breaking my lease, my father had acted on a belief that I was as good as dead.

I said nothing, but kept sipping my tea. Mom left the room. When Dad and Ramanan Uncle woke up, I confronted Dad, who quickly told me that it was the best thing he could do at the time. I said nothing.

Later that week, Ramanan Uncle left for Texas, while Mom, Dad, and I moved back into their four-bedroom, two-story redbrick Colonial house, nestled comfortably in the state in which I may have been born, but where I had no intention of dying: New Jersey.

I immediately went to the garage to find my stuff. When I saw all of my possessions stuffed into sealed cartons in the cramped garage, I was too stunned even to cry. All severe-brain-injury survivors suffer some sort of amnesia and must look through their personal possessions to regain their broken identities. I wanted that ritual of soothing recognition.

When I finally had the courage to open every box, I saw my journals, clothes, books, compact discs, videotapes, private letters, photos—and I realized that Dad had already seen and touched everything that I ever owned, and stuffed them into cardboard.

I said nothing.

In the Name of the Father, the Son, and the Holy Piss

Three days after I returned to New Jersey, one of my father's buddies, who lived in India, named Jignesh, invited my parents and me to visit him in Long Island, where he was staying for a weeklong business trip. Mom was feeling sick and exhausted, so Dad and I went alone.

In the middle of the rather long drive, I had to use the bathroom. As we drove into the parking lot of the next service station, we saw large crowds pushing into the cramped space. It looked less like a rest area than a bustling suburban shopping mall.

Dad joined me as we pushed through the human traffic into the men's room, which was situated way in the back.

The men's room was rectangular, gray, and shockingly clean, except for the standard pornoglyphic graffiti. Dad and I walked to the only two empty urinals available. They were next to each other.

As I began relieving myself, I realized the resentment I still harbored for my father. Why would he take away the home I had made for myself? How could he be so cruel to his own son? At age twenty-five, this apartment was all that I really had. It's odd how the most powerful feelings emerge while showering or excreting, but that is what happened as I stood pissing away.

"Dad, why did you do it?" I asked abruptly.

"Not now, Ashok." Dad knew what I was starting.

"Tell me, what satisfaction did you have removing my entire life?"

"I'm not going to discuss this right now," Dad murmured. "Are you mad? People can hear."

I masked my fury with a polite nod. "Fine, we'll discuss it later."

"You had all this time, and you pick a public restroom to talk about the apartment removal? What's wrong with you?"

I was furious. What's wrong with *me*? This man took away my home and he's asking what's wrong with *me*?

"Fine, we'll talk about this outside."

"Correct," he responded sternly.

Done pissing, after nearly two minutes, Dad appeared. He

had a habit of admiring himself in public restroom mirrors, so his late arrival, though irritating, was expected.

I looked at him, in his Rockport Slip-Ons, sky-blue dress shirt, and brown slacks. His face was worn, his spectacles dirty. He looked very, very old.

"Why, Dad?" I blurted. "Why did you take away my apartment?" I could hear the urgency in my own voice.

"It's complicated," he answered immediately.

I had entered a state of near combustion. "I'm listening," I said, with forced calmness.

"When you had the hemorrhage, nobody knew what to think. We were told you would be okay, but the full prognosis was unclear."

"You didn't think I would survive?"

"I didn't know what would happen to you. Neither did the doctors."

"But Mom had faith, she knew I wouldn't die."

"How could she! None of us did! I did the only smart thing to do. I closed your place up because we didn't know when or if you'd come back to us."

"I can't believe this!" I was getting very loud. "Why couldn't you have just stopped all electricity and phone services but still kept up the lease?"

"It was costing a lot per month. You know that. And with your future unknown, it made no sense to keep it. I had to think of the money."

"It was all about money, pure and simple? You know the doctors said I would need to see photos and personal materials of my life so the amnesia wouldn't increase!"

"Ashok, there were many complicating factors, but naturally the financial situation was at the top of the list."

"But how could you not be there for Mom? Seems you were too busy cleaning up my home to be in the hospital with her."

"She was in a dreamland. She wasn't thinking practically; one of us had to handle the finances."

"She was alone, so alone. She needed you in the mornings as she sat down by my bed, in the afternoons when she visited the chapel to pray, in the evenings while she sat alone eating in the dark cafeteria."

"I had a job, Ashok."

"But I feel now that most of your time wasn't spent on your job, but trying to find a maid to clean my house, and to get movers to take all my stuff into your garage."

"What are you talking about? Of course I was doing my normal job! But you have a point . . . I focused on closing up the apartment. It was a big enough job itself. It made sense to deal with it."

I paused for a moment, tears welling.

"You saw everything in my apartment."

"Well, I had to, since we were moving you out."

"You saw everything."

"Yes, I did, and everything's okay."

"How can you say that? I'm just twenty-five! Did you want your parents to see all your private stuff at that age? Or even now, do you want anyone to go through your private stuff?"

"You're right about that," he admitted with a sigh.

I was still horrified. My memories were quarantined in stacks of bland cardboard boxes. I had things to hide from my parents, like empty vodka bottles and stacks of porn. My father had gone through all of those things in clearing my apartment.

Dad spoke bluntly. "Bottom line, Ashok—I didn't know how or if you would make it through this."

Dad rubbed his eyes. "Forgive me for getting rid of that place." He continued, "But as they say, what's done is, well, done. We'll find you a new place, don't worry."

I didn't want a new place. I wanted my home back.

I didn't forgive Dad that day. But as the weeks continued, I finally did. I came to realize that by packing up my home, he was able to escape the real-life terror of the hospital. He could concentrate on his son's existing belongings rather than on the possibility of his son not existing at all.

He was my dad and I loved him, no matter what. And I would never stop loving him, no matter what.

But that day, as we sped off to Long Island, neither of us wanted to speak, so we combated the glaring silence by listening to the radio. I was surprised by how well Dad could sing along to Beyoncé.

Mom's Tears

"I killed you."

Mom's words awakened me.

"What?" I asked groggily, looking up at her. I was surprised to see her. She rarely entered my bedroom, but she was now near my bed, her flannel kaftan brushing my wooden bedpost.

I quickly located my eyeglasses on the dresser next to my bed. She appeared exhausted, her cocoa skin sickly, pale, and gaunt. Under her eyes were near-black blotches.

I looked at the alarm clock next to me. 10 a.m. Good thing she came, I thought. At least I wouldn't oversleep.

But looking up at her, I immediately remembered her awful statement. I questioned her once more. "What are you talking about?"

"I said, I killed you."

"Mom," I said, laughing, "the bhaji last night was awful, but I can assure you that I'm still alive."

She knelt down and held me tight. I could feel her tears as she hugged me.

"Mom, I don't know what drug you're on, but I promise I'm breathing. Nobody killed me. I'm still here."

"Ashok, I ruined your life. I'm to blame."

I could barely understand her as her continued weeping muffled her voice.

"I gave you the AVM. I destroyed your brain. I destroyed your world. I destroyed your life."

Her crying became louder, the sobbing unstoppable.

I squeezed her closer to me. I began crying too. "Please don't say that, Mom. You heard the doctor, it was a congenital defect. You had no control."

"Exactly. It was not genetic, it was congenital. That tangle grew in my womb. Heredity or not, it grew in my womb."

"But—"

"But nothing. I will always know that my body destroyed you. How could any mother do this to her own child! Dear God, what have I done?"

"Mom, stop. I made it through this. It's okay. What happened had to happen, but it's not your fault. You never drank or did drugs or anything like that! This was just a quirk of nature."

"Ashok, there will be times you won't feel that way. You will hold it against me, and you have every right to."

"Mom, that will never happen! I love you too much."

I hugged her tightly. Still weeping, she left the room, her hands over her wet face.

Unfortunately, as always, Mom's words would prove correct.

In time, the blame game would explode.

• • •

Baby

Because my death—and new birth—occurred on one fateful day, *March 17*, I decided to celebrate it as a second birthday every year. I even dubbed the milestone *Birthin' 2: Electric Boogaloo.*

By this new calendar, I had not even turned one yet. So I had a lot to learn, a young lifetime's worth.

It required strength, courage, patience, and a paradoxical combination of resistance and surrender, but like many survivors, I was damaged but still alive. Death had already visited, and he no longer scared me.

Yet evidence of the full extent of the damage caused by my hemorrhage kept manifesting itself. It began with my legs—they started to hurt severely. Two orthopedic doctors reassured me that after being in bed for many months, my legs weren't used to supporting my weight. I was ordered to take it slower, walking just a few times daily until the limbs adjusted to my weight. In addition, the left side of my body had become weaker from the hemorrhage, so I was made to lift tiny weights to strengthen myself.

I had become one of those old crones in adult diaper commercials. But somehow, I was prepared for that. Maybe it was because I knew every episode of *The Golden Girls* by heart.

The body aches were accompanied by severe headaches. The doctors said that continual headaches were normal following brain surgery, but I had no idea they would be so painful. They always made me think of just-opened potato chips: *crispy*. Yes, the headaches felt crispy, as if my skull's insides were being snapped apart, ready to be bitten and chewed by sharp, hard, pointed teeth.

Unfortunately, it also felt as if the teeth were already in my head—the potato chips were being snapped and broken right then and there. I just wanted to scream and pass out.

I was supposed to record my headaches on a number scale from one to ten, ten being the most excruciating. It was pointless—I always had "tens." I was advised to take aspirin. My stomach couldn't tolerate it, so while my head throbbed, I also felt constantly nauseated.

My sweet and gentle brain had been partially destroyed, violated, and torn. How could I be resentful while it fought back? If it had to punch and kick the membranes within my skull, so be it. It was allowed to misbehave. And I could only cry from the pain. Sometimes, two or three Motrins would provide relief and calm the tantrums of my inter-cranial baby. Usually, though, the inner problem child kept on abusing me.

The daily drugs began to deplete my energy. Some mornings I couldn't even wake up. If I did, I was so exhausted that my only activity was sitting on the sofa and watching TV. I created a name for this type of day: High Fatigue Day, or "HFD." On an HFD, a gravely weakened Ashok emerged—like a tiny bit of earthworm, squirming, after being cut off from its larger self. Cut off, but still living.

I used to look healthy, strong. Now, I was skeletal, broken. Cheekbones, once protected with fleshy chubbiness, were now bony protrusions jutting obscenely from each side of my face. Nausea and exhaustion had rendered my body ineffective in fighting off the pain and fatigue. On HFDs, my mind now had trouble simply adding two and two.

Adrift

Besides weakened legs, headaches, and HFDs, I soon discovered there were other painful consequences of the AVM bleed: a severe loss of spatial relations. Even before the hemorrhage, I would lose my sense of direction easily. Maps confused me; I was always quick to ask a passerby for help in finding my way. Yet I was still able to get around. Now, my sense of direction had vanished completely. North, south, east, and west were just words to me. When I ventured out alone, I would often get lost in neighborhoods I used to know well.

This handicap took center stage when Juan, a friend from Chicago who was concerned about my condition, came to visit me in New Jersey. It felt great to have him in our isolated home. The first day he arrived, he took me on the bus to New York City so I could show him my old haunts. We were planning to see Washington Square Park—the campus of my old college, New York University—after I showed him the Chelsea neighborhood of my previous apartment. The first part was easy: from the Port Authority bus station at Forty-second Street, we simply took a cab to Chelsea. After ambling through the area, we only had to walk a few blocks southeast to reach the park. But I had no idea how to get there.

"I know where we're going," I told Juan with feigned confidence. "Can't wait to show you where I went to school," I said.

"But we've been walking around in circles for the last twenty minutes," Juan protested.

It must be a wonderful spectacle, I thought: *one oblivious tourist walking with one oblivious brain patient down the streets of Manhattan.* I usually had no problems asking for directions. This time I couldn't bear to. After all, I had gone to NYU for four years, and I had worked in the area after that. I'm not that stupid, I thought. After searching for the park for thirty minutes, Juan and I finally returned to the bus station.

The next day brought a similar experience. Juan and I went to New York City for a meal at a renowned Lower East Side dive restaurant. After lunch Juan went to stay with a relative. That meant I had to return to Port Authority and then get back to Jersey—all of it alone.

My departure gate at the Port Authority was 435, located

on the fourth floor. I reached what I thought was my gate and walked through the door, which closed swiftly behind me. There was no bus, only trash cans: I had entered the garbage area. I panicked until I located another door that allowed me reentry.

My spatial difficulties were also evident in my trips to the movie theater back in New Jersey. I had to remember the location of the restroom in relation to the auditorium. My movie partners—usually my parents—would always help me find my way. *When you leave the theater, make a right, then a left, and then another left. Then you'll see the men's room. Come back using the opposite directions, right, right, left.* When they offered such instructions, I would nod and say thanks. But deep inside, my pride was hurt. Not because they were wrong, but because they were right: without their directions, I'd easily be lost.

Different Sounds, Same Semen

Tinnitus is the term for ringing in your ears and head. Temporary tinnitus can be caused by anything from waxy buildup to high blood pressure. But permanent, large-scale tinnitus is caused by severe damage to nerve endings in the ears. You always hear inner whines, high squeals, or even police sirens. And even worse, there's no cure.

I didn't know about the condition at all. When I was alone, in complete silence, I heard sounds. *What's happening to me,* I would ask myself, consumed with panic. *The television and every appliance is off, the family's gone out.* Still, I would hear the buzzing of swarms of bees, a high-decibel stereo, and even some distant ambulance siren. The trouble was that they were all inside my head.

One time I was sitting in the house and the noises grew particularly loud. I cried out to Dad, sitting in the next room.

"I can't stop the noises! Help me stop them!"

"What noises?" he said, rushing into the room.

"You don't hear them at all?"

"You should quit listening to your music so loud. It's messing with your ears."

After two or three weeks of ceaseless noise, I made Dad take me to an ear, nose, and throat specialist.

Dad and I nervously waited in the outer room. I thought about what the doctor would say. My mind strayed to the worst health scenario: perhaps another tiny hemorrhage had occurred. To distract myself from growing worries, I picked up *Highlights,* the kiddie magazine, and read the cartoon Goofus and Gallant. As an adult, I now found it oddly sadomasochistic. *Why would Goofus put up with that abusive shit from Gallant, unless it turned him on to be a slave to his friend? And why would Gallant seem to get hard every time he hassled Goofus?*

The doctor finally ushered me into his cramped, wood-paneled office. A tall, lanky white man with surprisingly full lips and darker than black eyes, he resembled, oddly, a black female model. He was a white, transgendered Iman.

He listened to my concerns and then directed me to what looked like a recording studio, where his nurse fitted me with oversized headphones. I suddenly felt like Prince, singing eccentric rhymes in his all-lavender studio in Paisley Park.

The nurse went to a separate room and began speaking softly through my headphones. She asked me to repeat some words. She sounded like a phone-sex operator, seductively purring random words like "SSSensssational" and "Mmmissing." Was I supposed to echo her, or get aroused?

After the tests, which I thought I had passed easily, I returned to Dr. Keele's room. Dad was already sitting there.

"Here's the reason for the noises," Dr. Keele said. "Ashok has lost half his hearing in the left ear. Could be from the meningitis or the brain surgery. His head has suffered so many traumas, it's impossible to say."

"Will he become deaf?" Dad asked.

"Not a chance," Keele said.

Dad looked relieved.

"There's only one problem. The damage to your left ear is extensive. The hearing will never come back. The noises will stay forever. It's called permanent tinnitus."

I said nothing, more than a little disturbed by the ongoing discoveries of internal damage.

Dr. Keele tried to offer encouragement by giving me coping methods to block out the noises.

Here were his three "Tinnitus Treatment Tips":

1. Don't be in quiet spaces.

2. Converse a lot.

3. Just try and ignore it.

I thanked him for his help.

Dad and I drove back to the house in total silence. That is, except for the ambulance siren still screaming in my head.

Masturbating had made my brain explode. So for a long time after, I was afraid to play with myself. However, after two months of living in New Jersey, I decided to go for it.

There was just a little problem: I had no idea if I liked boys or girls after the hemorrhage. This might seem ridiculous, but it was completely true, a very frustrating predicament. You see, a guy has to be attracted to something to get him aroused, and I didn't want to be asexual. So I gave myself a test to see which gender would get me hard. I looked through my parents' magazines for the closest thing to porn. I found two candidates: a *Victoria's Secret* catalog and *Men's Health*. I went to my room, took down my pants, and got to work.

I completed my mission. Twice.

To my surprise—and excitement—both did the trick. Nothing had changed from prebleed Ashok. Not that it mattered. Aside from pleasuring myself occasionally, I had little sexual interest. The brain bleed had ended that, at least temporarily.

The Wonderful World of Therapy

In order to exist once more, I had to do extensive therapy. You name it, I was doing it: speech therapy, physical therapy, occupational therapy, and most important, cognitive therapy. My brain bleed had left me with the brain of a newborn. I wanted to become an adult again. I sought teaching aids to stoke my intellect. I remember being given crossword puzzles to solve, and a test about matching people to occupations. That test was positively racist: the WASP guy was the lawyer, the Chinese woman was the violinist, the black man was the basketball player, the Indian guy was the engineer, and the Latina was the maid. I went on a tirade about prejudices and racism, a tirade which, while over the top, a least proved to the therapist that my intelligence was intact.

I was also progressing in physical therapy: walking, moving my hands, twisting my shoulders. I knew I was lucky, because many brain hemorrhage survivors become paraplegic or quadriplegic. That thought depressed me.

One of the exercises involved touching the middle fingers of my left and right hands to the tip of my nose repeatedly — a traditional exercise performed by drivers suspected of drinking too much. I was good at that one. I was also made to walk down a corridor with my head held erect and while keeping my balance, like a hallway Naomi Campbell on a catwalk.

Amid all the excitement of therapy, I joined a gym. I

always hated gyms, since exercising in front of buff people was humiliating. But this gym was actually a rehabilitation center frequented by senior citizens. Seeing eighty-year-olds attempting squats made me feel better about myself.

On my first visit to the gym with Mom, I felt weird. My arms were in bandages and I still had my head wrap. As we reached the center, a lady was walking in. She was bowlegged and hunched over. When I came to the front desk, I saw that she was the check-in person.

"Hola!" I said, trying to seem casual, but trying too hard.

With a sigh, she told me to sign in.

I stared at her. She was more than bowlegged; the left side of her face was paralyzed, a mask of pink concrete. She smiled but her mouth could open only halfway. I smiled in return.

"Have you had brain surgery?" she asked me.

"I guess my head wrap gave it away," I said.

"My skull was opened, too," She said. I looked closer. She appeared to be in her early forties, skinny and very Caucasian.

"I had an AVM bleed and a craniotomy," she said.

At that point, I yelled with glee, probably stopping half of the hearts on the workout floor. And then I hugged that hunched, disfigured woman. I had finally met someone like me!

"What's your name?" I asked.

"Carol."

"I'm Ashok."

We hugged once more.

I never knew recognition could feel so good. At that moment she became my sister, a member of the family. Her body was damaged in the same way as mine. Our skulls had been opened. All brain patients were now related to me.

I would never see Carol again, but it hardly mattered; having met her in the first place was good enough for me.

Warning: Memory Lane Under Construction

Having once considered amnesia a plot gimmick used only in soap operas, I now realized it was real.

I began to take inventory of my memories. I could barely remember important life events from after the age of twenty. I could barely recall anything of the week leading up to the hemorrhage. While my memory slowly improved, I learned I was suffering from more than amnesia.

I had completely lost *emotional* memory. I could intellectually remember places I had once frequented. For instance, when I finally found Washington Square Park—thanks to a map and a passerby—I could recall my NYU days. But the memory invoked no feelings. My heart remembered nothing at all, even though I knew I had been there. Frightened by my lack of emotions, I did a quick experiment. I phoned my mother, asking what she remembered about giving birth to Prakash. I wondered if she would recall more than the date.

"It was surreal, magical," she said.

I said, "That's great—but can you actually experience those feelings right now, as you mention the day?"

"Of course! My heart feels warm just thinking about it. And I'm smiling."

I subsequently asked Prakash and Dad similar questions about important events in their lives. Both responded similarly, recalling what they actually felt in the past.

My short-term memory was destroyed. Since I couldn't remember what another person had just said, I was unable to sustain conversations.

Once, Karmen and I were discussing the 2000 presidential election.

"Can you believe Bush stole the election?" she said.

"Not surprising," I agreed, "since Katherine Harris was already backing him up, serving as his oral glory-hole in Florida."

"Definitely. Now we have a fake president in the White House. What do you think about that?"

I hesitated and looked at her quizzically. "What do I think about what?"

These types of conversations would happen all the time.

I used to try to laugh it off, explaining that I was having "senior moments," until I realized there was nothing funny at all. The short-term brain fizzles weren't confined to conversations; I couldn't watch video movies without hitting the "pause" button, since I already would have forgotten the previous scene. Moreover, I would forget characters and dialogues within five minutes. In the movie theater, I was no longer able to enjoy a film.

Eventually, after watching public-access television programs about brain boosting, I discovered an exercise to strengthen my short-term memory. It involved Prakash.

He would have to write a list of random words and then read the words to me. I was to repeat those words back, correctly. With my cognitive skills barely evolving, I never fully succeeded. Example:

Prakash: "Red, Coma, Wednesday, Technicolor, Morphing."

Me: "Red, Coma, Windy, Testicle, Mormon."

I tried to bulk up my retention skills by watching game shows, focusing on the quiz questions and the puzzles.

I became hooked on "Wheel of Fortune," forming, in my mind, a warped, virtual-reality ménage à trois with Vanna White and Pat Sajak. At first, I would be unable to solve the puzzles, let alone remember the categories. Eventually I became an expert.

Still, improvement was slow, reminding me of the extent of the damages. This was not science fiction; my brain really had detonated.

Not even Vanna could have prevented that.

Jeepers Creepers, Where'd You Get Those Peepers: 2000 (VI)

Learning from Marilyn Monroe

My vision therapist murdered me and saved me at the same time.

A proudly femme white man, Walton was six foot four and weighed only one hundred thirty pounds. In a breathy voice suggesting a Marilyn Monroe drag act, Walton confronted me about the issue I had tried to avoid: my half-blindness. The doctors had already discussed it with me, as had my parents, many times. But I had not intellectually understood the condition. There didn't appear to be a cutoff point in my vision, so I believed it was completely intact. It took a while for this to sink in, because Walton's Monroe accent was so distracting.

But no matter what distractions I faced, I still had to learn to see. My sight had been cut in half, down the middle—in both eyes. The AVM had burst in the right side of the back of my head, the location of the occipital lobe, which governed sight. The hemorrhage had left me half-blind for the rest of my life, a condition called "bilateral homonymous hemianopsia."

But there had been a problem: although the doctors told my family that I had become permanently blind on the left side as soon as the hemorrhage happened, I, myself, was never informed of this during my incarceration, as they feared this news would be too great of a shock to my system—and might damage any chance I had for a sound recovery in the hospital. It was only after my release that the doctors and therapists felt it was safe to inform me that I had become half-blind. It took Walton, however, to nail it into my head.

Not only had I become blind in the left half of each eye, but I had a blind spot near the middle of my field of vision.

Walton taught me how to compensate for the vision loss, how to turn my head back and forth to widen the field of vision and rapidly shift my eyes from side to side while my head was stationary. I resembled a 1930s screen villain, mustachioed and shifty-eyed, ready to trick detective Charlie Chan. I was told always to stay on the far left in group situations, in order to see as much possible. Walton told me to do this every time I was in public, from concerts to jogs to movie theaters.

Ole!

It was difficult to adjust to my newfound vision loss, as I quickly discovered. The first time Mom, Dad, Prakash, and Karmen took me out to eat, we went to a family-oriented Mexican restaurant with sombreros and street signs on its stucco walls. On the Friday night we stepped out it was fully packed.

We were given an unnecessarily oversized booth. As Walton had instructed, I sat on the left end, far removed from the others. Mom sat near my right, while the others sat on the facing side. Our waitress was a pretty white coed, who, judging from her accent, must have been a recent transplant from the South. Her name tag said KATHY-KATE.

"How y'all doin'?" she asked after we sat down. Her smile was warm and inviting. "I'll give y'all a moment to look over the menu."

When Kathy-Kate came back, she asked which drinks we wanted. Everyone ordered Cokes except Mom, who specified "Sprite, with no *ice!*" (It's been my experience that many Indians are obsessed with drinking ice-free liquids.)

Since it was my first time out, I celebrated with a virgin strawberry daiquiri.

We placed our orders when she returned. I chose the three-chicken enchilada platter, while the others ordered equally standard Mexican cuisine.

Some time later, Kathy-Kate returned with the food.

We dug in. My family became involved in an animated conversation, leaving me on my own. It felt like I was on a football field yards away from the action, but I was happier that way, since I had overheard snatches of their discussion, which that night centered on Rosie O'Donnell.

After nearly fifteen minutes of slowly consuming my tasty enchiladas, rice, and refried beans, I noticed my food quickly vanish. I was puzzled.

"Hey," I muttered to Mom, reaching to tap her shoulder. She didn't pay attention.

I spoke much louder, and tapped again. "Hey, Mom."

She seemed irritated to leave her conversation.

"They didn't put much food on my plate!" I yelled. "Look at it, where are the enchiladas?"

She finally turned toward me. There followed a ten-second silence.

"Oh God."

Upon hearing her cryptic statement, Dad, Prakash, and Karmen stared at me.

"Your pants," Mom gasped. "Look at your pants. And turn your plate around."

The left leg of my light tan cargo pants was greasily coated with a pungent mess of two smeared enchiladas and a splattering of wet beans.

I spun the plate from left to right.

Sure enough, the left side was bare. I had only eaten from the right section of the plate. As I had no vision of the left side, my fork had speared the rest of my meal off the plate and into my lap.

I looked at the damage without saying a word.

Dad yelled for Kathy-Kate, who had lost her earlier charm completely by ignoring us throughout our dining experience.

"Excuse me!" he boomed, "Kathy-Kate, we need your assistance!"

Smiling as if she never left our side, she walked to the booth.

"How's everything, Shug?"

"My son has made a bit of a mess. We need some extra napkins and some more water."

Her eyes widened at the sight of the mayhem.

"No!" I yelled defensively as the other patrons watched. "I'm fine, I can clean this up!"

"But there's a lot of food there, Shug," Kathy-Kate said patiently. "I'll be back so we can clean this in a jiffy."

"Fine," I said in resignation, surveying the damage my blindness had created.

She came back with paper towels and water and that old stand-by, club soda, to mop up, of course.

I had to wipe my lap myself. I doubt she wanted to come near my bean-and-salsa-soiled crotch.

When we left, Kathy-Kate received a hefty tip.

A Different Kind of Video Game

Reading, writing, and making art were three of my most vital prehemorrhage activities. I feared that the vision loss would render them impossible, so I started to work to restore my skill. The first book I attempted to read was from the Harry Potter series. I did so with a ruler, placing it under each line of text so I knew when to move to the next one.

It took me a week to read it. When I finished, I had never been so happy to follow the adventures of a four-eyed moron.

I learned to write again by choosing random subjects, like celebrity substance abuse. Whitney Houston became my muse. I wrote my epics in no time, without errors.

Creating art, though, was a problem. I used to love symmetry in both my paintings and drawings. My favorite subject was portraiture. Now that I could not see half a face, I worried that I would never paint again. "Picasso went through many phases of art during his life," people reassured me. "This is the new shape of your art."

The resulting faces, rendered in acrylic paint on canvas with the help of rulers and grids, looked far from human. My first large-scale piece was called "Self-Portrait: Damage in Utero." It depicted my mother, completely nude, her uterus visible. Inside was embryonic Ashok, his young brain bleeding. I submitted "Self-Portrait" to a New York City gallery show called Terrorvision. It was rejected.

My vision rehabilitation involved seeing a neuro-ophthalmologist specializing in brain-sight issues. The doctor's name was Ferdinand Damore, and he was fantastic.

Named one of America's leading neuro-ophthalmologists by a popular New York magazine, he was a short white man with glasses whose lenses seemed thicker than his legs. Walton referred me. I knew I was lucky to have Dr. Damore, although I always wondered why a top eye doctor resembled Mr. Magoo.

At every appointment, he made me take a "field test," perhaps the worst exam since the SATs. This was like a Playstation on smack. I had to look through a telescopelike instrument, viewing a large, empty gray screen with a sunlike object in the middle. Stars of all sizes, from large to minuscule, moved across the screen. Every time I saw a star, I had to press the button on a joystick.

It was meant to measure my field of vision. But every time I did it, I knew I couldn't see a star on the left side unless it touched the sun. I had to take the test multiple times. Each time it was over, the doctors presented a printout of the actual field, with dots indicating how many times I saw the star. Each time the result was the same: one side was covered by dots, the other side was empty, confirming a lack of vision, straight down the middle, in both eyes.

I tried to justify my vision loss. *The world was bad enough with perfect 20/20; I'm lucky that I can witness only half of it.*

Or I reminded myself that the left side was historically the "sinister" side, so I was free from evil. But these were feeble attempts.

The vision loss was insidious: there was no white or black line—or anything for that matter—to indicate where my vision ended. I thought I saw everything in my field of vision, when in fact, I was only seeing half. Although I wished I could see fully again, I began to understand that my situation would likely never change.

I was told I could never drive again. Taxis and buses became my new best friends, the subway my soulmate.

My hemianopsia reinforced the emotional amnesia that was occurring in my relationships. Rather than simply forget general feelings about past experiences, I would also forget short-term fighting and reconciling. Say I had a fight with someone in the morning, and we made up in the afternoon. We're friends again by evening, laughing and joking. The next morning, I remember we battled. But I don't remember the resolution, or how I reacted. Upon waking, my anger is fresher than ever.

Poor Prakash had to deal with this memory roller coaster often. Especially concerning my sight loss.

Day 1
11 a.m.:
I'm talking to Prakash on the phone.

"Ashok, I have some interesting news for you," he says, sounding both delighted and smug.

I'm getting excited. *Interesting news? I love interesting news!*

"I can't wait to hear it, Prakash, and don't spare any details."

"I'm getting a new car, and I'm really thrilled about it. I can't wait to drive it!"

"That's great, have fun in it," I say glumly. After a moment of silence, sound returns.

"You don't seem too happy about it," he complains, "if it was the other way around, I'd totally be happy for you!"

"Fuck off," I say. Then I hang up.

11:10 a.m.:

Prakash calls back. "Why did you just do that?"

"You do realize that I can never drive again, right?"

"Oh please, nobody believes you're really blind, you're probably faking it. You look fine."

"Why would I lie about this? I would give anything to have my sight back! I don't want to take buses forever."

"Just think," Prakash says, laughing, "now you can join the losers, cheapskates, and ex-cons who always take public transportation. It'll be fun."

"Karma's going to bite your ass. Not only will you wake up blind, but you'll be paralyzed so the only way you can move is in a wheelchair."

"Whatever," he says and laughs again, easily dismissing my comment.

"Don't talk to me again, asshole, until you learn how shitty it is not to be able to drive!"

"You're such an idiot, I'd love to not drive for the rest of my life. Let someone else have that job!"

"Then why did you sound so excited about your new car? Obviously you wanted to get behind the wheel."

"That's true." I heard the glibness in his voice. "I *am* excited to drive it! You're so smart!"

After yelling at him to stop calling me, I hang up again.

6 p.m.:

Prakash calls me as I'm getting ready to watch *King of the Hill*. The silly all-day fighting exhausted me, so I thought a little cartoon fun would cheer me up.

"I'm sorry, bro," he says. "That was insensitive. I realize you wouldn't lie about your vision."

"I told you not to call me back."

He sounds serious. "I said I'm sorry. I'll make it up to you by getting you a great dinner when you next come to my place."

"Just promise to understand how I feel about losing part of my sight."

"Of course I will, let's move on."

Day 2

7 a.m.:

The ringing phone wakes me up, half an hour before my alarm clock is supposed to wake me.

"Hello?"

"Ashok, it's Prakash."

"What do you want?" I respond aggressively.

"Just wanted to say good morning. I got you upset yesterday, so I wanted to check up on you."

"You jerk! How can you talk to me this way?"

"What the fuck?"

"You don't even remember? You made fun of my blindness, asshole!" My voice level rises. "I'm your own brother, and this is what you say!"

Every nucleus in me is freshly angry. All I know is that I hate my brother for not only gloating about his new car, but doubting my sight deficit in the first place.

We reconcile, once again, that afternoon.

This Groundhog Daze of fighting, resolving, and refighting usually lasted four days or so. Then, finally, I would move on.

Day 4:

I call Prakash in the morning, and in my sweetest voice I say, "I'm so happy we're friends again!"

"Asshole," Prakash responds, hanging up.

AVM Wha . . . ?: 2000 (VII)

Dr. Evil

He resected the AVM!

He untangled the bruised veins and arteries!

He stapled titanium clips to the ends of unattached blood routes!

He screwed in the metal plates to put my skull back together!

His name was Dr. Fennet.

Conventionally handsome with close-cropped black hair and extremely tall at nearly six foot four, he had pale ochre skin and looked like Michael Jordan struck with anemia.

It can be argued that he saved my life. After all, one clumsy cut and I'd have been in a wheelchair for life, or forced to learn sign language, or forced to move with a red-striped cane.

As I fought for my life, Dr. Fennet was the surgeon: the main man whose hands held drills and knives to my skull and navigated through the bloody swamps of my brain tissue.

He had performed the thirteen-hour craniotomy.

He done good.

Over time, my mind had gained strength. I wanted to immediately remember all I had forgotten: college days, the job I had once had, family members. I had started to read about brain surgery; I wanted to know what had been done to my noggin.

Like a traumatized adult trying to remember childhood abuse, I begged for answers. My parents said they didn't know. *There has to be some record,* I argued.

Now we were finally going to see Dr. Fennet, months after my hospital release. I was thrilled; I could finally ask what he had done to my brain. I had all my questions written precisely in a small red spiral notebook. I had rehearsed them with my folks, in the car all the way there.

We were finally called in. My parents and I took turns hugging Dr. Fennet, the man responsible for my second chance at life.

He sat in a black leather swivel chair behind his desk. We sat across from him in red plastic low-back chairs. He checked the back of my head, did a quick test of my eyes and nose, and was finished. It took all of ten minutes.

He looked suspiciously at the red notebook on my lap.

"Doctor Fennet," I started, like an eager junior high nerd, "I have questions for you regarding the surgery."

He cleared his throat, as if preparing for the acid he was about to spit in my face. "No need," he said.

My face fell. "What do you mean, no need?"

"I mean, it would be counterproductive for me to tell you."

"I have no memory about what happened. You were the surgeon who operated on me! You have to tell me," I pleaded.

"I will not tell you," he replied in the same flat voice. "You would never understand, even if I did."

This had to be a joke. How can the man who put his hand into my skull not have any info for me? I almost began to cry.

"Look, you're fine. You're in good shape. Thanks for coming."

Dad intervened, demanding, "Tell us how many metal clips are in his head."

"Two, maybe three."

"You don't know exactly?"

"It was so long ago. Go get a hospital report if you have to. I can't find Ashok's file anyway."

There were more horrifying comments to follow from my so-called savior. Among them:

"I went to many years of medical school to learn about AVM resections—why should I tell you?"

And then:

"I have performed countless surgeries like yours. What makes you so special?"

And finally, the coup de grace:

"I'm the man who saved your life. That's all you need to know. Put your pen away."

My parents and I stood up and stormed out.

"Look," said Mom, breaking the silence as we drove away, "Like he said, he saved your life. That's all that matters. Who cares if he didn't have all the answers?"

"Who cares?" I exploded. "I do! How would you like to lose a hip and not know how it happened?"

We resumed the silence and it lasted the entire drive home.

We later contacted good ol' Prithvi, our relative from Canada. He urged us to obtain the operative report.

I took the next step: disgusted, I wrote a scathing letter to Fennet's boss, the head of neurosurgery at the hospital. I was still jolted. Why would Dr. Fennet behave this way?

To get the ever-elusive operative report, we had to contact the hospital's chamber of files, fill out applications, make appointments to meet a neurology director, etc. I'm surprised we didn't have to breakdance in the hospital lobby. When it finally arrived, I was newly distraught; it was hard to understand—and my very own surgeon should have fucking explained it.

Drunk with Success: 1992–2000

Phi Beta Kappica Alcoholica

NYU introduced me to other Indian Americans. But after attending eighteen years of Midwestern tractor pulls, I had little in common with them. Again, I became part of a reassuring gang of misfits.

This time, however, we misfits had a home base: nightclubs.

Yes, the drug haven—debauched, multigendered, multisexual. Places where I could wear my hair in devil horns, clump around in huge platform boots, and meet sexy boys and girls.

Even though I went out almost every night, I never took drugs or alcohol during college. Being the unapologetic nerd that I am, I felt that since it was illegal, I wouldn't dare take those substances.

In 1996, I graduated magna cum laude and Phi Beta Kappa, with a B.A. in Journalism, minoring in Philosophy.

I then decided to go to graduate school at Columbia University for the South Asian Studies program. The scholarship I had been offered was very inviting; besides, I had absolutely no clue as to my future direction. Why not study my own heritage? I figured.

Life at Columbia wasn't that great. Classes were filled with conformo drones, unlike the lovely individuality that sparkled in NYU. I learned nothing, really. I also found myself forced into being the token representative of "Indian American culture." After a few semesters, I quit.

It was now time to make up for the years I never drank while in NYU, which I did in a big way. I became an alcoholic.

It started with drinks after class. Then drinking in restaurants with friends. I favored the occasional vodka-cranberry over ice. Soon, one cocktail became two, three, four and five. Not just at restaurants, but everywhere. Eventually I was knocking back nine drinks on school days.

In the mornings. Before class.

I liked the way I felt when I drank my mixture of vodka and whatever. Drinking was very satisfying. When I first guzzled it down, I became hyper, friendly, and gregarious. But eventually, like all drinkers, I became contemplative, emotional, and sad.

When the sadness hit, I usually would be in a club with friends. At some point, after several drinks, I would wonder if I should stay and party, or go home and watch the movie

Titanic. I loved the sorrow drinking caused. The *Titanic* tear-fest would usually win.

But as the habit escalated, I looked around me and realized I had no idea where my life had gone. I fell into a deep depression, continued drinking heavily, and entered what I felt to be a future without meaning. And remember, this was before my brain exploded.

Liquid Public Relations

In late 1997, I found a job through an ad in *The New York Times:* "Renowned public relations firm seeks an enthusiastic junior account executive." Sounded exciting and promising. After making it through a stopover in academic hell at Columbia, this seemed like the path to now follow. So, being desperate, enthused, and most likely drunk, I immediately applied.

Luckily, as I soon found out, public relations was a great place for an alcoholic, as the business not only welcomed drinking, it demanded it. I got the job and kept on boozing.

The company I entered was called Steven Karter Public Relations, a top New York City firm.

I learned so much at SKPR and got two promotions during my stay there. My clients included global corporations, musicians, fashion houses, and filmmakers. The CEO, Steven Karter, called me a "star," and even invited me to his ultra-expensive Upper East Side townhouse.

As I started working there, however, I immediately began to understand ABM, or "angry black man," syndrome.
Simply stated, it is a term that means society always has to
watch out for black men, who are always "ready to attack."
It also means something a tad more insidious: black, or in
my case, brown, men are tolerated only if they "remember
their place." If men of color actually try to be assertive,
and—god forbid!—succeed, we are immediately dubbed as
"arrogant" or—in the case of a term recalling historic racism
to blacks—"uppity."

Well, this brown boy became well-versed in this dynamic.
I traveled up the proverbial ladder rather quickly, moving
from junior to senior account executive in the course of a
few months. While acquaintances—people of color—would
compliment my success, I found many of my white coworkers would dismiss my achievements. Walking past the conference room, unseen, I heard a gaggle of (white) coworkers call
me names that expressly implied that I was less than humble.
Of course, I took this as all part of the job. As a non-white
man, I had learned this was to be expected.

After all, I reminded myself, men of color who behave as-
sertively are "arrogant."

White men who do the same are "go-getters."

That mattered little though; I continued doing my job,
and a week after the boss invited me to hang out in his apartment, he asked me to play golf with him and his buddies.

This, of course, was the worst crime of all. A brown man playing golf with his boss, as if he were rising in the ranks? Afraid of the consequences, I turned him down. But, over-looking the expected racial issues pertaining to the job, I was doing good work and actually enjoying my time there.

Of course, not everything was perfect that way—the sin-ister, inebriated side of my life always showed its shadow. My hardcore drinking was escalating. I drank: at home, with friends in clubs or bars, and, of course, at hip parties. What made my alcohol abuse even worse was that I was succeeding at my job, which entailed approaching journalists and pro-ducers to guarantee client exposure. I was good at this. Very good. Plus, many of the journalists I contacted were drunk anyway. Drinkers love other drinkers.

I would get totally plastered at night, but unlike others, I could no longer claim the renowned metropolitan classi-fication of "functional drunk." I couldn't awaken early the next day. More frequently, I was calling my assistant in the morning to announce that I wouldn't be in until 3 or 4 p.m.

When I finally arrived, however, I worked my ass off, and had the media placements to show for it. Within a few weeks I got clients featured in *Time*, *Newsweek*, and *The New York Times*.

I awoke every single morning with heavy-duty headaches. I assumed these were routine hangovers, and dealt with them by simply swallowing plenty of aspirin before heading to work.

My behavior soon became erratic: I would yell at cowork-ers, forget phone calls, enter meetings irresponsibly late. But my bad behavior was tolerated. I was a PR hotshot, so no one ever said anything.

On one chilly spring morn, I was supposed to attend a press conference at the United Nations, launching a global fundraiser. I had to be there at 9 a.m.

My alarm went off at 6:30. Considering I had hit the pillow just an hour before (after a night with buddies in an East Vil-lage bar), I pressed snooze. Thankfully, I woke up, by accident, at 7:45.

I had set out my charcoal gray Tommy Hilfiger suit. (I was too poor to afford any other designer.)

After putting on a random white shirt (maybe Fruit of the Loom), I donned a red Versace tie (my budget allowed for higher-end ties).

So, there I was, garbed in a lovely charcoal suit and red tie.

Now, I am extraordinarily hirsute, and even though I shaved the night before, I had ridiculously thick, unruly morning stubble. I wanted to keep my face smooth, but there was no time; unshaven I went.

The last problem: to deal with the liquor smell that wafted from my body.

I located the cheapest, bargain-basementy cologne I had in the bathroom and showered myself with it.

When I arrived at the press conference, I was luckily just ten minutes late. What transpired is a haze, I'm afraid. All

I remember is the smelliness of the cut-rate cologne. So did everyone else. I overheard one older white man in an untailored suit lean over to his friend, and ask:

"Do you smell that?"

"The stench coming from that young man?" his friend replied.

"Obviously. It's the same smell from the cab I took to get here."

"Do their people *ever* bathe?"

That press conference continued smoothly, but my drunkenness did not, causing similar problems in other major events as the weeks progressed.

After working in the firm for nearly one year, I decided to leave. In my hazy, clouded mind, I believed I was not being paid enough for the great work I was doing. It was an alcohol-fueled decision, but a decision nonetheless. In my exit interview with Ling-Yu, the sexy, Trinidadian office coordinator, I was still a little drunk from the night before, so I couldn't help but ask a question that had been haunting me ever since she joined the company.

"Ling-Yu," I asked, "why do you have such an East Asian name?"

"My parents conceived me while watching Chinese porn. Ling-Yu was the name of the actress in it."

She looked up, dreamily. Then she turned to me, suddenly. "Ashok, do you know what's been happening here?" she whispered.

"No, what?" I said, thinking that she was going to tell me how the coworkers couldn't stop discussing how "arrogant" I was. Even better, I was wondering if she was going to tell me that the partners were planning a surprise farewell party. I was wrong, on both counts.

"Everyone says you've been on drugs all the while you've worked here."

"Huh?" I didn't know how to react. My mind was still scrambled a bit—the residual effect of twelve Jack-and-Cokes from the night before; however, her next comment was like a pot of black coffee.

"They say you're on those fancy designer drugs from all your party-hopping, and I'm not supposed to tell you."

You gotta be shitting me, I thought. At that moment, I was so fucking happy to be leaving that den of dirty gossip that I had never even considered the ramifications of what had been said. Besides, they had incorrectly assumed I was on "designer drugs," when it had been cheap vodka all along.

My "morning" headaches were now occurring all the time, even on those rare mornings after a sober night. Instead of heeding their warnings, I dulled the headaches with barrels of aspirin. But then I had no idea of what lay ahead.

Only a Few Days to Go

A headhunter found me a spectacular new opportunity: a job as account supervisor at Lennox Publicity, a smaller but impressive PR firm. I had my interview with the CEO, Jon

Lennox, in the company's offices, a spacious, hardwood-tiled suite with open cubicles instead of walled rooms.

When I arrived, a tiny, grumpy East Asian receptionist with platinum Jean Harlow hair told me she would call Jon over. I sat on one of the arty crimson chairs in the waiting room, sectioned off from the main office by a large cactus.

The first thing I noticed when I first saw Jon was his bright, oversized floral shirt, the type of shirts worn by guys who video girls getting nude on spring break. Baggy green cords finished his look.

He was white and slight and over forty. Barely five foot five with a pigeon-gray crew cut, he had tiny shaving cuts on his upper lip, which meant he was clumsy. Always a good sign in a boss.

"Ashok Rajamani?" he said, unexpectedly pronouncing my name perfectly. "I'm Jon Lennox."

I was volcanically trashed, having drunk nine whiskey sours just thirty minutes before.

Bathed, once again, in nearly a full bottle's worth of trashy cologne, I didn't wear a suit but rather a rumpled black T-shirt over a dirty white long-sleeved thermal tee, stained muddy brown from weeks of unwashed use.

Trying to regain my composure after relaxing on the red seat, I stumbled when I stood up to shake his hand.

"Heya man! Cool to meet you buddy!" I exclaimed.

This was the way I greeted the person who would be my senior boss.

Looking surprised, he smiled and walked me to his huge "work area." I was enraptured by the silkiness in his feathery voice. It was welcoming and relaxing. After some casual talk about the weather and VH1, he asked for my résumé.

I didn't pay attention to whatever he said after he perused my one-sheet. I just kept nodding my head, and when it seemed I was supposed to say something, I said variations of "I'm a work in progress" and "public relations is my life."

Embarrassed by my drunkenness, I felt horrible as I looked into his kind eyes. I was betraying and fooling an innocent person, so rather than focusing on the conversation, I was concentrating on whether or not he knew of my self-saturation.

Before I knew it, the interview was over.

He hired me on the spot.

Only at Lennox for a week before my brother's wedding, I was barely introduced to my coworkers and received no paycheck before taking the plane to Washington, D.C.

Big Apple Core: 2000–2001

Oy Vey!

While I was hospitalized, Prakash had been having weekly phone talks with the CFO of Lennox. The CFO had decided that when I returned to the firm, my workload would be drastically changed. Before my surgery, I was working from 9 a.m. to 6 p.m. On my return, my workday was shifted from 10:30 a.m. to 4 p.m.

But that didn't matter. I was just fucking thrilled to be able to come back to work at all. It had been four months since my hospitalization.

Although my apartment was gone, my city wasn't, and I wanted to be back there, in the center of the world, living alone, living without the parents, living life.

But was it safe to leave home? Mom and I decided to check with my medical gurus. We asked one of my neurologists.

"Ashok has done enough therapy. He is perfectly fine to live on his own," he said.

His reassurance satisfied Mom, and I was given permission to move to the city, leaving my parents with a nest as empty as the one I had abandoned years before, when I had first zoomed out of Illinois.

The hunt was now on to find myself a home in New York. I had to find a place in Chelsea. Since I had lived there right before the bleed, it would be easier for me to make sense of the city; my reassimilation into urbanity wouldn't be as difficult as if moving to an entirely different locale.

Plus, Lennox's offices were in the heart of the neighborhood.

My fury at my father for giving up my apartment had intensified. *Why must I even deal with this,* I thought. *My home should still be there, I should be concerned only with regaining my health, not regaining real estate!*

And so began my daily, relentless reading of the *Times*'s classified section, as my parents and I looked for names of realtors offering rental apartments.

Finally, after our fingers were bleeding black ink from constantly scouring the newspaper ads, we discovered the apartment of my dreams. The realty company name alone sold us: Oy Vey Realty.

That was definitely the right name. Nothing else came close.

CHELSEA: *Small one-bedroom apartment. Freshly painted and sparkling. Great closets and storage. Lovely tree-lined setting. Walking distance to subway stations. Immediate occupancy. One-month security, one-month fee. No pets. Unbelievable price.*

Dad called the number listed with the ad, spoke to a charming lady, and made an appointment for the three of us to visit the company's office, located in midtown Manhattan.

When the door opened, we were surprised. Instead of the harried Jewish spinster we expected to meet at a realty company called Oy Vey, we saw a cheery Indian woman. She was under five feet tall and adorably plump. She greeted us with her tiny thick hand, adorned with pricey gold bling.

"Hi, my name is Oviya. Oviya Raman."

Dad recognized the voice from the phone.

She began laughing. "I'm the owner of Oy Vey. Get it? Oviya . . . Oy Vey . . . same sound, no?" She was laughing. "Get it?"

Dad and I politely smiled. The four of us left her office and cabbed it to the apartment, which, sure enough, was on a lovely tree-lined street in West Chelsea.

There, in front of the small four-story walk-up, we met the landlord, Isa, a rather short, solidly built, olive-skinned middle-aged man, with an epic mustache.

"I'm Isa, the landlord here," he said. He was wearing a T-shirt that said I HONK FOR HOOTERS.

Dad shook his hand and beamed, enjoying the man's thick

foreign accent. He was always delighted to find another soul who bludgeoned the English language as much as he did.

"Isa, are you from India?" he said. "We are too, we came from Mumbai."

"No, sir, I am from Cairo, been in States for nearly five years."

Dad smiled. He liked this Isa fella.

"Let me show you the place," he said.

His tour consisted of him waving his arm toward the living room and bedroom, much as the models do when showing prizes on "The Price Is Right." There wasn't much to show, obviously, as it was a tiny place as advertised. But wow, was it sparkly, clean and freshly painted! The ad was telling the truth! I couldn't help but feel pride as I looked at the shiny coral walls. So clean, so fresh, and soon to be all mine. True, the place had a minifridge in lieu of a kitchen, a wee bathroom and a bedroom smaller than an office cubicle, but this was to be expected.

The price was great, affordable enough for Dad, who was going to foot the bill until I got back on my feet. Most important, it was located just blocks away from my work.

Without hesitation we snapped it up, and offered to sign for it immediately.

Unexpectedly, Mom exclaimed, "It's too soon! He's not recovered!"

Dad was calm. "You heard what his doctor said; he is in perfect shape. We have to let him go."

We bid Oviya au revoir, went back to Jersey, and signed the necessary documents over the next few days.

My meager possessions, which had been removed from the cardboard boxes, were now stuffed back in. Movers took them from Jersey to my new apartment. The cartons didn't bother me now: I had officially forgiven Dad.

I finally moved in three weeks later, giddy to be independent again. Barely five months after brain surgery, and I was moved into my new apartment in the city. I had just turned twenty-six, and this was the best birthday gift imaginable. Content, I began to immerse myself in the new environment. As I unpacked my books, CDs, clothes, and the filthy-cheap futon, I started to make my house a home, to paraphrase that lovely song.

Unfortunately, it took just a couple of weeks for the sparkle and shine to dull. I found mice, I lost heat, and had to bathe in frigid water.

This was my new home, though, and I didn't care how irritating the conditions were. So what if I had a few problems? Happens all the time. I would get accustomed to wearing coats in the living room, and as for my furry friends, it was nice not to be so alone.

Now that I was back in my homeland, I began to question my existence, and my resurrection. Being a former Baby Buddha, I recalled the Buddhist concept of Nirvana—the ecstatic, final liberation and annihilation of body, self, and ego. My legendary namesake, Ashoka, the famed Indian emperor, was responsible for the largest global propagation of the faith, spreading its teachings throughout India and Asia.

I wondered if he'd be proud of me. After all, I had been annihilated . . . or at least my body had.

Perhaps I had already reached Nirvana, if only for a teeny moment.

Not really, of course, unless Nirvana meant unwanted vermin and an arctic apartment with freezing water. Baby Buddha still had a long way to go.

Accidents Do Happen

"Watch where you're going, asshole!"

"Ouch muthafucka!"

"Jerk! Why'd you just knock into my friend?"

My ears ached with every nasty comment. I was far from the safety of Jersey; I was now back in New York City, which meant weaving through the crowded streets, tasting the rank core of the Big Apple.

In addition to being able to live on my own again, I was thrilled to have another welcomed revelation: my lust for alcohol was over.

When I first left the hospital, I was terrified my liquor addiction would return. In New Jersey, I would tell myself, *let's try to stay sober this week, and then go from there.* I needn't have worried. As the days passed, my love affair with booze faded. The intense desire that once consumed me was gone, and as days went on, I stopped thinking about the sauce. Soon, my ex-lover didn't even enter my mind.

After three months of nondrinking, I was finally unchained from the monster.

Looking at my reflection in my new flat, I spoke out loud: "Ashok," I said, "it's over."

My reflection looked doubtful. Skeptical bastard.

"Ashok, you're free. No more Smirnoff, no more Absolut, no more Jack Daniel's. They are out of your life."

The reflection gave me a reassuring smile, but he remained doubtful.

More time passed. I had absolutely no longing for the hard stuff—straight or on ice. My white-trash side no longer craved vodka mixed with Snapple Lemonade. I had absolutely no hunger for the excitement or, more important, the sadness, alcohol gave me.

When I confronted the mirror again, my reflection was no longer doubtful. I was free.

Because of this excitement in being completely sober, having my own Manhattan apartment again, and being independent and back in my hometown, I forgot Walton's training. Funny, one would think I'd never forget the holy lessons of the Dalai Walton, who taught me the art of handling half-blindness. But how could I remember, when I was listening to my iPod and bopping down the street to the latest Coldplay download? So yes, I began bumping into people. Even though half the world was missing, I thought I saw everything.

The verbal assaults, though, were nothing compared to the physical bumps. Well, more than bumps. Two cars hit me. The first time was at Union Square, when I was following a group of New Yorkers walking against the DON'T WALK sign. I thought I was safe in the group, but I was at the back of the pack. A man in a blue Mercedes was fed up with the jaywalkers and hit his accelerator. I didn't see him, but I felt his car slam into my left leg. When I turned my head to see what happened, all the way around, swiveling like an oscillating fan, I saw a spot of red welling up under the denim on my left leg. The driver looked at me angrily, believing that I stood there intentionally—that I wanted to get hit. It was my first run-in with an automobile, and a valuable lesson: never walk carelessly through Manhattan, half-blind, humming a pop tune.

The second time it happened, I was crossing Fifth Avenue with the permission of the green WALK sign. But I didn't count on New York cabbies. I felt a bump. Then I heard two folks scream loudly from the sidewalk, "Holy shit! That dude just got hit!"

They were talking about me. I looked down and once again saw blood on my jeans. Then I looked up. It must have been a hard collision since the cab's headlights had been broken. I was frozen with fear.

Out came the cabdriver, short and rotund. Sepia-toned

with a pencil-thin mustache, he shouted, "Leyyet me take you to the hyospitayll! Pleayaz I will get you help!"

Jeez. He's Indian. Figures.

The man spoke pitch-perfect South Indian English. He begged to take me to the hospital. Maybe he was afraid of a lawsuit. Or maybe he was just a decent guy noticing that he had hit a brutha.

I told him that I was all right and walked away. But when I got to the sidewalk, I started weeping.

An even worse incident happened days later. I woke up from deep sleep with an upset stomach and urgently needed relief, so at 3 a.m. I sped off to a nearby Rite Aid to get crackers and ginger ale. Chelsea was oddly quiet, with relatively few pedestrians. As I swiftly ran through an empty, random street, I smashed into a tall metal post firmly planted at a sidewalk.

I was thrown back to the unclean concrete from the sheer force of the collision. Getting up, I didn't think anything of it, and speedily tried to walk home, even though my head throbbed.

But my face felt wet, and I tentatively touched it, fearing the worst. The fear was validated. My hand was covered in blood.

I held my forehead with my hands and ran blindly for help. A deli clerk directed me to an emergency hospital up the street. I got there in a couple of minutes, shoved my credit card into the nurse's face, and was eventually sitting in an examination room with a kind doctor.

After carefully inspecting my blood-dripping forehead, he asked me a question.

"What drugs were you on?"

"Nothing, nothing at all," I said. "I was just running and didn't see the pole." I could tell he wasn't convinced.

"Well, you have a massive, massive cut. Looks like I'll be giving you stitches, probably around twelve. But don't worry, they'll be in your eyebrow area, so your handsome face won't be scarred."

I blushed. "Thanks for the compliment."

Then, as if the Pope himself had just entered the room, he whispered to me conspiratorially.

"Seriously, what drugs were you on?"

The Comeback Kid; or, Any Publicity Is Blind Publicity; or, I Still Don't Remember Walton

Beyond dodging maniac cabs and murderous street-light poles, I faced a more terrifying challenge: going back to Lennox PR.

My quick reentry into the workforce — mere months after my skull had been opened — was approved by my crack team of medical professionals, the same experts who had already given me the go-ahead to be a lone citydweller.

At this point, my home life was becoming fantastic. Isa was actually taking care of the problems in my new apartment, and I was in perfectly livable conditions. No more mice, no more winter coats indoors.

Arriving on my first day back to work, I spotted my boss at the lobby elevator. "Hello!" I shouted, too loudly. I hugged him tightly; I had become overemotional since the surgery. He gave me a salute and an awkward smile.

We shared the elevator ride in unnerving silence, and when the doors opened on our floor, everything looked different. I barely remembered the faces that greeted me, but, because of the brain bleed, I had no shame in hugging everybody as I had Jon, since, after all, I had become basically a slobbering puppy.

Although I was excited to come back to the offices, I hadn't anticipated how my half-blindness would affect work. But during one cold week in February, I found out.

On Monday, my coworker Rosa asked, "Ashok, is something wrong?"

I was cheery, and had no idea why she was looking at me odd. The next day, another coworker, Blaine, also spoke to me quizzically: "Your face . . . Is everything okay?"

I ran to the bathroom. Didn't have snot running down my nose. No zit under my eye. What's he talking about? I thought. For the remainder of the week, I kept hearing the same chorus from my coworkers, all confused by my appearance. Days after, I would scream at my assistant, Helen. She was a lovely Cuban-American girl who smiled at all the employees. Why would I be yelling at sweet Helen? I wasn't drinking anymore.

But I displayed a growing frustration with her. One specific incident proved it. One day, I was checking a random spreadsheet. "You missed the addresses, Helen. This is the third time! What's wrong with you?"

"What are you talking about?" she said, her patented smile fading for the first time. "Everything has been done."

"Why were you even hired? You are incompetent!"

Helen walked away, furious.

A couple weeks later, while visiting my parents in New Jersey, I went to a Sharper Image store in a mall. I wanted to treat myself to an expensive high-tech gadget, to celebrate my return to the workforce. *Maybe one of those massage chairs. Or a nifty cell-phone holder,* I thought. Instead, I found a three-angle mirror, the kind found in clothing store dressing rooms, except this wasn't a full-body version.

I purchased it. When I reached my apartment, I ran to the bathroom and set up the mirror on the sink.

I screamed.

The morning's shave had left one side of my face covered in cuts. My sideburns were completely uneven. One sideburn reached mid-ear, the other just scraped my chin. One half of my face was blotched with blood.

I had unknowingly become both monster and victim of a slasher film.

There and then, I understood.

All this time, I hadn't been able to see that part of my

face. I wasn't aware I was demolishing that half every morning. Now I understood Blaine and Rosa's comments, their horror, and why they were staying away from me.

I must have been a living cartoon—probably working the half-moustache look, too. For the short time I had been back in Manhattan, no one had been close enough to me to be honest about my appearance. My parents were no longer right there with me. I had no roommate, and after the hemorrhage, I had lost contact with the handful of close friends I once could claim. Even the good stitch doctor had said nothing, perhaps thinking the marks were simply a result from the pole injury.

I also figured out that smiling Helen had not screwed up; I just couldn't see the far left portion of the spreadsheets.

In the end, I realized this was all my fault. Just because I wasn't walking into people on the streets didn't mean my sight had returned. Once again, I had forgotten Walton's teachings.

Still, nothing, nothing at all, could completely dry the tears that fell every time I peered into my three-angle mirror.

White Editor Likes Her Magazine Color-Free

Before work every day, I looked closely into the dreaded three-sided mirror. Multiple times, if I had to, to ensure that I was clean-shaven all the way around, no half-and-half. To make life easier, I no longer maintained sideburns.

It worked; coworkers stopped staring at me. And now I

scanned the entire spreadsheet to confirm Helen's work. Her perma-smile soon returned.

But I still had to deal with the intellectual deficits caused by my exploded brain: deficits that created a humiliating back step in my professional career. My boss was a stern forty-something white woman, who selected me to rep a popular high-end magazine catering to fortysomething women. She took me to meet the magazine's well-known editrix. Since it wasn't a corporate confab, I wore a simple blue button-up shirt and black slacks.

The magazine's headquarters was an intimidating space, commanding an entire floor of a prominent New York City skyscraper. Hardcore WASP women walked the halls. I had never seen such a concentration of blond hair, cardigans, khakis, and sensible shoes. They all looked as if their idea of heaven was Cape Cod. They could have been Martha Stewart clones, but weren't—they seemed too cheery.

My boss and I walked down a long hallway of these Cape Coddesses, and were shown to a room that contained steel chairs that resembled bar stools for dwarves. In walked the publisher, an imposing woman, white, tall, and brown-bobbed. She was in standard Hamptonian drag: relaxed brown slacks and, yes, a very Martha beige cardigan wrapped around an expectedly pristine white turtleneck. We sat at a large, rectangular glass-topped table.

"I'd like to introduce Ashok Rajamani, who's going to work for the magazine," my boss said.

The publisher sighed, obviously underwhelmed.

"Oh, hello," she said dismissively.

"I'll do a fantastic job," I exclaimed. "I'll get you media exposure *everywhere.*"

"Oh yeah?" she said, her face stony.

As it was extremely early in my recovery, and my mind was not yet at full speed, one ridiculous thought came to mind: Everyone wants to be young and hip. That's modern, that's what's salable!

"I'm going to present you as young, hip, urban, and modern," I announced proudly. "We'll get all the readers we need!"

"Are you serious? That's not our demographic at all," she barked. She looked at me as if speaking to an incompetent.

I had nothing to say but "Um . . . Um . . ."

My boss sat quietly as the publisher systematically grated me into sienna-stained shreds.

"Thanks for your time," the editrix snapped abruptly. She was sneering behind a smile.

"It was nice to meet you."

She stood up. The meeting was over.

The next day at work, my boss called me to her office.

"Our editor friend called," she said. "She's thinking of leaving our firm. We definitely *cannot* lose this client."

"Oh wow. I'm sorry."

"She gave me the reason, Ashok."

"I think I know it already."

"She told me, 'How dare that kid not wear a suit to the meeting!'"

I gulped in disbelief. "But what about the foolish things I said?"

"It wasn't brought up. The main thing was that you didn't fit the 'look' that best represents the publication."

"Meaning?"

"First of all, she wants a woman. Second, she thinks you might look too . . . um . . ."

"Ethnic?"

"NO!" she shouted, and then looked down sheepishly. "She thinks you're just, well, a little too *urban*. But I told her you were a sensational publicist, and that you could do a great job."

"Thanks . . . I guess."

A week later, we had a second meeting with the publisher. This time, a coworker, Jane, came with us: a preppy white blonde girl wearing the regulation WASP uniform, cape of khaki cardigan included. Her costume aside, she was an adorable girl, always lovable, kind, and sweet to me. We sat again at the glass table and prostrated before the Queen.

My boss spoke first, sounding artificially cheery.

"Great news! We have a new person to handle your account."

We fucking do?

"Her name is Jane. Ashok won't be on the account."

I was officially fired from the account. In front of the client.

Back at the office, my boss cooed to me in her sweetest tone, "You understand that the workload is very heavy for someone of your, um, condition."

I didn't know if the condition was my pigment, or my brain. Turns out it was the latter, as she pointed to her head, nodding gravely. Before she would be able to kick me out, I gave her my two weeks' notice. Her expression was confusing. She said nothing, but gave me an odd half-smile. I couldn't tell if she was happy to be rid of a brain-damaged employee or viewed my resignation as the welcome removal of a dark stain on her snowy-white firm.

It didn't matter, though. I didn't request a recommendation letter.

Time to Bloom: 2001

Beach Indian Bingo

Freed from my public relations job in January 2001, I laughed, I sang, and cried official tears of joy.

I entered a new era.

I started exercising. Until now, I had never even enjoyed walking. My binge drinking had left me bloated yet puny, my body a collection of fat and bones. But I had lost the excess weight after the brain bleed, along with any muscle I may have had.

Now I began running on a treadmill. And while I ran, I listened to power ballads on my CD player. I even sang along with the ridiculous anthems, such as Des'ree's "Life." They were hokey songs, but inspirational for someone who had cheated death. "Life, oh Life, Oh life . . . doo doo doo doo," she belted. And boy, did my tears fall. I couldn't help crying while I ran, singing that schmaltzy "doo doo doo" with gusto. I put that song on repeat so often that I eventually destroyed the CD.

On my off days I unwound with less-than-inspirational songs. "Dying" by Hole was an example. As Courtney Love droned, "I'm dying, I'm dying please," I sang along in grave self-pity, all the while taking a philosophical approach to my life. Granted, my singing was bad, since I had just learned to hum once more. But it didn't matter. In my mind, I had become both Preacher and Riot Grrl.

In August of that year, my parents celebrated my survival by taking me to Aruba for a holiday. The reason for this trip was rather simple: it was a mother's promise. During my hospitalization, when I fought through the crushing pain of the drillings in my skull, needles in my skin, and tubes through my nose and throat, my mother would say to me: "Ashok, if you live through this, you will never have to see metal again. Just trees, sand, water, and you will have seaweed wraps!" As silly as it sounds, her promise helped to give me the strength to withstand the daily hospital nightmares. I never, ever, wanted to see anything metal, or steel, or plastic, or any such material around me again. I only wanted trees, sea, sand, and all forms of nature. When Mom would make that daily promise, I would shut my eyes tight and dream of seaweed wraps. I dreamed of flowers of rainbow hues and plants and soft sands. I dreamed of swaying trees. And I dreamed of all the colorful seashells I could ever hold. These dreams were partially responsible for keeping me alive as I lay restrained in that dark, scary hospital room.

My mother kept her word; here we were going to, of all nature's paradises on earth, Aruba! I was so excited that I went shopping for my first bathing suit. I found a bright green baggy one in a low-end suburban department store, along with flip-flops and some towels.

The trip began with a tremendous headache. En route to Aruba, I experienced a number nine on a scale of ten, which required my popping some Motrin. As I looked out the window, I saw that everything down below seemed to be painted in vivid colors. When we landed, my father ran to the information counter where we were told that our bus was running half an hour late. Typically, he yelled at the workers, flaring his nostrils and swaying his hips.

There is a great Indian family tradition of waiting in airports, mainly because we book extended flights that entail long stopovers. During this ritual, the mother or grandmother eases the children's impatience by feeding them dry foods—usually pistachio nuts—saying "Beta, Kalo" ("Son, eat"). Why this is a tradition, I'll never know. So, like a good Indian family, we waited in the airport. My father, wearing his too-tight white T-shirt and matching shorts, kept looking at his watch. I wondered where my pistachios were.

"Calm down," I said. "It's not as if we're late for a meeting."

"Humph!" he retorted, petulant as always.

When the bus finally came, we were taken to the hotel we were staying at, the Aruba Royale, an old-fashioned place whose lodgers had a median age of sixty. No matter; since the AVM I liked quiet environments, and this place seemed to offer it in spades. We stayed on Palm Beach and had it all to ourselves. Before we arrived, I had already decided I would only swim at night. Being partially flabby and morbidly hairy, I had no intention of letting the world see me topless. But that changed when I went to my parents' suite.

My mother had changed into a bathing suit—a sleek black one-piece with a pink racing stripe. *How could she, in daylight?* I thought. Just when I was recovering from the shock, my father appeared, topless and hairier than I. That does it, I decided! If they could do it, so could I. I'm going day swimming too, without a top!

It turned out all my fears were pointless. The beach had a European sensibility: The men had hair on their shoulders and backs. The women had tits hanging to their calves. No body-conscious people in sight; they were all topless.

I was pleased. We should all live as God intended us to. I wondered why America—and the Brazilian wax community—didn't feel the same way.

Shameless in our lack of clothing, my parents and I relaxed in lovely white plastic lounge chairs. The sun hit our mahogany skin, turning it darker than the darkest of chocolate.

Stepping into the ocean was one of the greatest experiences of my life. I slowly realized that this is why I didn't die — I had yet to live a life like this, free and alive. If nothing else, my near-death experience had given me a new appreciation of life, and of all the wondrous things I had taken for granted.

Yes, Virginia, There Is a Terrorist. He's Every Brown Person in America.

Six months after our Aruba trip, Mom and I decided to make a brief return visit. We arrived in paradise, once more, on September 9, 2001.

Two days later, we had just come back from the beach to our hotel room when Prakash called.

"We're under attack!" he said. "Turn on the TV!"

We watched in horror at the events that were unfolding back in my city.

As a result of the attacks, we were stranded in Aruba for five extra days: no planes were allowed to leave or enter the U.S.

Dad used his frequent-flyer miles to secure us first-class tickets home. When we boarded the plane, we had no idea what was in store for us. You see, we didn't know that all of the 9/11 terrorists had been in the first-class section. When we took our seats, everyone stared. To make matters worse, Mom had wrapped her black scarf around her head like a cloak—only because she was cold—making her look like an orthodox Islamic woman.

And then the fun began. When I got up to use the toilet, four flight attendants quickly surrounded me. "Can we help you?" the quadruplets asked, failing to camouflage the panic on their faces. When I didn't answer quickly enough, a blond male attendant—whose Teutonic vibe would have made the Führer cry with joy—joined the circle. Everyone in the cabin was watching intently—except Mom, of course, who was sleeping all snuggled up in her makeshift burqa.

As I scanned the flight attendants around me, I felt disgusted. I responded—as loudly as I could—"Yes, you can definitely help me. All of you can hold my penis for a while and then shake it. I have to pee."

They lowered their faces and silently slunk away. Unfortunately, this was merely a jarring preview of what I was coming home to.

As we landed in New York City, I looked out the airplane window and saw countless American flags waving at half-staff. My first response was not sorrow for my beloved country; it was complete dread for my family. I somberly looked at Mom, and said simply, "We're all dead, all our people."

I was right. Upon my arrival, Dad told me that a friend of his, a good-natured Sikh man around the age of sixty, was murdered while working the cash register at a grocery store. A thirtysomething white man, wearing an IT'S ABOUT FREE-DOM t-shirt, had walked up and told him, "You destroyed America."

Then he shot him in the face, point-blank.

We lived in fear from then on.

New York, like the Pentagon and that field in Pennsylvania, had been horribly scarred, but it was surviving. Like most folks, I was horrified by the terror attacks and the lives they destroyed. Now I faced potential harassment, even physical harm, within my own land. I had faith, though, in my dear country's resilience.

America had experienced the worst disaster of its life. It would survive. So would I.

Dancing and Singing and Praying, Oh My!

Twenty-six was an awkward age at which to have experienced death and rebirth. I had completed my education, but had barely established a career.

Since I quit the only professional world I knew, public relations, the prospect of a new career frightened me. I had no work experience other than manipulating journalists and TV producers to give my clients some media exposure, and, perhaps, no other skills.

I refused to go back to the unchallenging world of public relations. Not that I was a genius, but I could use my

resurrected brain for something better than promoting racist magazines and figuring out the inane codes of fashion
failures.

So I went to a career-planning workshop at NYU. Quick
testing revealed that my primary interests—writing and art—
blended sweetly in advertising. I was excited, foolishly believing that advertising was a step up from publicity.

Tanya was a friend of my sister-in-law who worked in
corporate marketing. Over lunch one day, she talked to me
about advertising. But first Tanya told me a bit about herself:
she was born in Sicily and had given up a child for adoption
at age fifteen. She had just left an abusive husband.

She told me to sidestep details about my brain surgery at
job interviews. This was a strong woman, I thought, who
could help me, and I could learn a lot from her.

Calling in a favor, she got me an interview at a leading
New York City advertising agency. I met first with the human resources manager. He got to the point immediately.
"In your résumé, there's a large time gap from the date of
your last job."

"There's a reason for that," I said, remembering what
Tanya had said about not divulging my hemorrhage. Another
friend, a business associate of Prakash, had told me simply to
lie. My parents' Indian chums suggested that I invent reasons for the gap in my work history, such as "I was traveling
around the world," or "I had to take care of my dying uncle

in India." My big bro and parents instructed me to simply say that I had had a health issue, and to leave it at that.

But I thought there was nothing shameful about my condition, and I intended to tell the truth.

"I had a brain hemorrhage, so it took all this time to fully recover."

"I see." Curt, non-committal.

"I had to learn to walk, talk, and even use the toilet again! But here I am, in fine shape!"

"Are you saying that your brain had some sort of damage?"

"Well, I'm saying that it did become damaged, and then it was fixed. And now, so am I. Just look at me!"

The HR man gave me a strained smile and became overly cheerful. "Your résumé looks great. I'll give your information to the creative director. Her office is next door, but she's in a meeting, unfortunately. She'll definitely call you to set up an interview. Thank you for your time, Mr. Rajamani." His lips were tight.

I wanted to curry his favor further. I asked what his sign was.

"I'm a Capricorn."

Grinning, I prodded him more. "So you must be dating other earth signs huh?"

"Actually, I'm getting married next month."

I asked what was his lady's sign, what kind of wedding they were planning, and was he going to have kids?

He quickly looked down at his wristwatch. "Mr. Rajamani, I should go now. I enjoyed speaking with you."

I was thrilled, he was obviously hurrying to the office next door to talk with the creative director. I sincerely believed that I had been hired. *I can't believe this! I got the job!*

Strangely, he had left his office before I had.

Leaving the building, I was ecstatic to finally work again. That weekend, I went to Macy's to buy ties and a belt, even though the purchases strained my current bank account. But what the hell. I would have a career again!

Two weeks passed. No word came from the creative director, no summons to her office. I called the HR man and left a quick message. Kinda ghetto-style, unfortunately.

"Hi, it's Ashok Rajamani. I haven't heard back from the director. Wassup wit dat?"

Not exactly professional, I realized, but only after I hung up.

Oh well, maybe he'll think I'm joshing him, that I'm considering him a homey.

I never heard back.

After going on two more job interviews, I finally learned to put a cork in the brain-bleed story. I had officially suffered an unspecified illness. If they pressured me, I would say "aneurysm."

While I was depressed by the lack of progress on the job market, I at least had my life back. Why look for the same job again? Life was, as I had realized, too fragile and too short for me not to consider new directions.

So I listed possible jobs that would give my life meaning.

1. Ballroom Dancer: I loved dancing and wearing costumes.
2. Talk Show Host: I could be a one-man currified version of *The View*, doing shows such as "How masala can drive your man wild" or "What to do when you catch your husband wearing your sari."
3. Recreational Director: Watching a pretty volleyball instructor in Aruba had inspired me.
4. Songwriter: I could certainly write any number of inspirational or sad tunes after my near-death experience, from uplifting Jesus-hand-me-a-ladle country ballads to sorrowful my-husband-left-me-for-a-crack-whore heartbreak anthems.
5. Priest: I loved God, and there were lovely Hindu temples in Queens—only a subway ride away.

Listing fantasy professions excited me. My future was wide open. It didn't matter that I currently had no income. Although physically I wasn't 100 percent perfect, I could see, hear, talk, and walk without cane or crutch. And I didn't need a wheelchair.

Still alive and with my functions fairly intact, I had been given another chance to relish the world, excluding the hell of public relations and including the heaven of tropical beaches. The world seemed to be mine, and I could grab it any way I wanted to. Such possibilities!

I had never felt so delighted to have survived my brain's explosion.

Just When You Thought
the Worst Was Over: 2002

Fear in a Handful of Air

Nothing is shocking; everything is shocking.

I should have realized this vital truth in my life, after all of the surprises and twists and terrors I had so recently undergone. I shouldn't really have been shocked by what happened following 2001—but I absolutely was.

On January 19, 2002, Manhattan was pummeled by a large-scale blizzard. At eleven that evening, my friend Ringo and I were heading to a late dinner. Ringo, named after the most underappreciated Beatle, was a young, handsome black man, my age and height, with striking shoulder-length ebony dreadlocks. On Seventeenth Street and Sixth Avenue, I started to feel ominously ill. It was an unfamiliar, magnified mix of flulike exhaustion, head pain, feverish sweating, and severe nausea. I had never before felt this terrible.

As the snow kept furiously bombarding us, I began shouting "Get a taxi!" to Ringo.

I needed to go home, fast.

Suddenly, I was hit with something greater than the severe sick feeling I had known before; I was now inhaling and exhaling a vile, invasive odor that seemed to envelop me.

If death had a stench, this would be it: a repulsive, unbearable combination of car fumes, melted gunmetal, and burning rubber.

Then blackness.

I awoke in a hospital bed. Déjà vu. The ceilings were mustard yellow. This time it was not Prakash looking over me, but Ringo. His mocha face was warm and reassuring.

I was more lucid than I had been after the wedding-day hemorrhage, and immediately I noticed I was again strapped to a bed. Next to Ringo stood a short, oddly oblong East Asian man who was more horizontal than vertical.

"My name is Dr. Lee. You're in Beth Israel's emergency room. You've just had a massive seizure, so we've hooked you up to a strong anticonvulsant, Dilantin."

Sure enough, my left arm was pierced with a huge IV drip.

"We don't know what might have precipitated the seizure."

I told the story of my AVM and the brain bleed.

"Ah," Dr. Lee said in reply. "That probably explains it. Let's give you a CT scan to see what's up." He led me from the room.

As I returned, by myself, to the bed, Ringo jumped at me. "What's your family's number in New Jersey? I have to tell them!"

I gave him the number, feeling as frightened as he looked.

Mom was by herself when she received the call. Dad was in Berlin on business.

"Mrs. Rajamani? It's Ringo. There's been a problem— Ashok is in the hospital!"

Having just nursed me back from the long, long road out of hell, Mom refused to accept another medical terror.

"Ringo," she scolded, "it's almost one in the morning. What an awful, disgusting joke. Why would you even say this to me?"

He gave me the phone, informing me that Mom wouldn't believe him.

I took the headset, and told her that Ringo wasn't joking. "Mom, it's true. I'm in Beth Israel."

"Oh my god."

"But it's all right, I'm okay."

"I'll be right there!"

Poor Mom. She was devastated, but fortunately, Prakash and Karmen were nearby, spending the weekend at a friend's home in Newark.

She called my brother, crying hysterically.

"Don't worry. Don't cry, and stay calm," he said on his cell phone. "We are coming right over—don't even think of driving to the city. We'll take you there."

As they were driving through the storm, Ringo told me about the events surrounding my arrival at the hospital.

It turns out that he was so panicky that when the nurses asked him for my information, he gave them wrong answers.

We were still talking when Prakash, Karmen, and Mom arrived, breathing heavily from their rapid trip. Shortly after, Dr. Lee arrived with his results. We looked at him nervously.

"Got some good news and bad news for all of you."

I hated it when people said that. It *always* meant they *only* have bad news for you. Adding the "good" is just to soften the shock. And it fucking never succeeds.

"The CT scan showed that your brain hasn't changed."

He paused to deliver the kicker.

"But the AVM scar has become a recurring irritant to the brain. It will provoke seizures from time to time. You're epileptic."

Furious, Prakash spoke up.

"Why did this happen after so long? Two years after the hemorrhage?"

Dr. Lee didn't even blink at my brother's angry outburst, but continued calmly.

"First, the surgeons were probably too concerned with the AVM brain surgery and keeping Ashok alive to discuss the risk of epilepsy. As for the long delay in having a seizure, it's a textbook case. It's called the 'kindling effect.' When the brain suffers a massive injury, it's as if a wildfire has been 'kindled' in the brain.

"After a long time, the flames—that is, the seizures—finally emerge. His hemorrhage left a scar. When it's irritated, it affects brain electricity, and Ashok seizes."

Dr. Lee looked at Ringo.

"Will you please describe, in detail, what happened during the night? We know it was a seizure, but I need to hear more specifics."

Ringo looked troubled, as if recounting the tale would hospitalize him as well. He sighed.

"No problem, I'll tell you."

Dr. Lee and my family leaned in closer as he began speaking.

"When Ashok and I neared the restaurant, he looked really sick, dry-heaving and all that shit. He started shouting for me to hail a taxi. I kept asking if he was okay, but he didn't respond.

"He got real clumsy, like he was losing his balance totally. Then his body . . . his body . . . changed. That's the right word. Changed."

"How, Ringo? How did it change?" Dr. Lee asked, the urgency in his voice betraying the calm he was attempting to convey.

Ringo stopped speaking, distressed.

"It's okay. Take your time, go at your own pace," said Dr. Lee reassuringly.

After a minute, Ringo continued. "Ashok's body suddenly

clenched up. Hands and feet curved into claws, like a crab. His body totally hardened and became bone-stiff and rigid. He looked like a skeleton, like a fossil. He started to drop to the ground."

Mom looked down, shut her eyes, and covered her face with her hands.

"I couldn't let him hit the ground, and it looked like nothing would stop him from falling. So I grabbed his body with both my hands. And I held him up so that he wouldn't slam into the concrete. It was frozen with ice, where we were walking.

"His body kept jerking and thrashing and moving. I was so scared. I never knew a human body could ever become like that."

Ringo's voice became soft.

"The only thing I could do was hold him tightly as his body kept on flailing. I needed to call 911 but I had to use both my hands to hold him. Then, out of nowhere, I saw this white chick racing up the next street. She looked like she was in a hurry, wherever she was headed.

"I yelled to her, 'Please help me and call the ambulance!' She was an angel. She used her cell to call 911. She told them what was happening and gave them the address. I thanked her, and she sped off, no names exchanged. I was still holding Ashok. I didn't know what to do because his dead weight was becoming heavier than I could hold.

"Luckily, just then another person walked up to us. A dirty, raggedy homeless man. Poor guy, looked like he was completely drugged out. He carried an old newspaper and told me to calm down, told me things would work out.

"Then he unfolded the newspaper, placed it on the icy street, and instructed me to lay Ashok down on it. Like he was making a bed for him."

Ringo choked up, forcing himself to maintain his composure.

"The guy had nothing but that newspaper. But he laid it down for Ashok. Within five minutes, the ambulance showed up. And the paper guy walked away.

"Two big guys, I don't know if they were firemen or what, tried to lift Ashok onto the stretcher and into the ambulance. But I couldn't believe what I saw. Ashok fought, punched, and attacked them. It took them five minutes before getting him in the ambulance and restraining him with straps.

"During the entire time they forced him into the van, he kept crying out the same thing, over and over: 'Help me God Help me God.'"

Mom still held her head in her hands as Ringo finished speaking. Prakash and Karmen were visibly shaken.

I was horrified.

I remembered none of this.

Finally, Dr. Lee spoke. "Thanks for telling us what happened, Ringo," he said. "I know it was hard for you, but you did a great job recounting it. And you saved your buddy's life."

Ringo nodded, attempting but failing to deliver even a small smile.

Dr. Lee then gave us a cold, clinical explanation of what had happened. The distance in his voice was unnerving.

Mom looked up, dried her eyes, and listened intently.

"Ashok experienced a 'tonic-clonic' seizure, commonly known as the grand mal. It is the most severe of such attacks."

Thatta boy, Ashok. Always getting the first-place blue ribbon.

"Tonic-clonics cause more fatalities than any other type of seizure," Dr. Lee continued.

"In a grand mal or tonic-clonic seizure, there are two parts. First, the person enters the 'tonic' state, where he becomes unconscious, falls, stiffens, and hardens completely. Second is the 'clonic' part, where he jerks forcefully. Then he becomes unconscious. This extreme, severe quaking is often too much for any body to tolerate, so these types of seizures frequently cause permanent injury. Or they simply kill."

Dr. Lee looked directly at me.

"Ashok, you should go back to Jersey and recuperate with your parents for a while. I want you to see an epileptologist there. I'm familiar with a great one named Dr. Silvie; she's over in Jersey City. I'm also prescribing these Dilantin pills; you have to take four daily for the next three weeks."

"Three whole weeks?" I said, surprised by the lengthy period.

Little did I know that I would eventually have to take anticonvulsants for months. Years. The rest of my life.

Dr. Lee wished me well and left.

After an hour, Ringo left for the subway to get home. It was still snowing around five a.m., when Mom, Prakash, Karmen, and I left the hospital. Karmen stopped first at *Casa Ashok* to pick up some of my belongings, before we headed to Jersey.

I thought I had found freedom in New York City, but obviously freedom didn't want me just yet. So back to the parents' home I went.

The next afternoon, Mom and I went to see Dr. Silvie for a referral for a epileptologist closer to my parents' home. A sixtyish white woman with an even whiter mop of curly hair, she was calm and patient. Although her words echoed those of Dr. Lee, she did provide unexpected, startling information about the air to which I was condemned, speaking rather formally for a woman who looked like she just finished baking chicken pot pie in her country kitchen.

"What exactly was that, that . . . I don't know . . . that odor around me, Doctor?" I asked. "It felt like it was being inhaled and exhaled simultaneously."

"It's called an aura."

"And all along I thought an aura was a good thing, beautiful cosmic energy, filled with rainbow colors," I said with a smile, trying to be funny, but instead sounding as if I still believed in unicorns.

She smiled. "In this case, it's a severe warning before a

seizure. It includes intense sensory alterations, frequently accompanied by an unbearable odor."

"So that was the smell."

"What you breathed was a signal that an electrical malfunction in your body was on its way."

"So much for my aura," I mumbled.

I Sing the Body Electric:
2002–Present

Brand New Deaths

Epilepsy. Epileptic. Not words I'd ever wanted to try on for size. I had always thought of epilepsy as something foreign, far removed from my world. Until now, for me it had only been a punchline from an episode of *The Simpsons* in which the cartoon family was watching a quick-speed Japanese anime flick. Suddenly, Marge, Bart, Maggie, and Lisa are on the floor, shaking uncontrollably. They are all having seizures.

The audience is supposed to laugh.

After my January 19 seizure, I wasn't likely to laugh at seizures anymore.

I quickly learned more about the world of seizures, and met the doctors, the epileptologists, who are committed to preventing them.

Dr. Silvie recommended we see Dr. Dobbins, whom she

insisted was a pro. Mom came with me to the office of this "pro." Dr. Dobbins was a fortysomething woman with an Irish brogue. Within one second of my having described my experience to her, she said tersely, "Can I speak to you alone, please?"

Wow, I must be dying, I thought. *My seizure must have been the first sign of a terminal illness.*

When Mom left the room, she pounced on me.

"Ashok," she said, as she paused threateningly. "Were you drinking liquor?"

Defensively, I responded, "No, I haven't done that since the hemorrhage. Why?"

"When you drink, you can cause a seizure."

"Not a chance. Didn't have a drop," I said, before pausing for a second or two. "Hey, why did my mom have to leave?"

She looked at me gravely. "Mothers should not hear about their sons' drinking."

You gotta be fucking kidding me.

From that moment on, I disliked Dr. Dobbins.

She prescribed more Dilantin. Three weeks later, I was alone in my parents' Jersey home, watching TV. They had gone to the city to see a Broadway show. The smell of burning rubber hit me again. It was another grand mal seizure.

I quickly ran upstairs to the bathroom, hoping mouthwash would rinse away the taste of hell in my mouth. It didn't work. I raced back downstairs to the fridge, hoping to find food that would kill the taste. I devoured chocolate ice cream. No luck.

Next thing I knew, I was on the kitchen floor, my legs shaking back and forth on the cold ceramic tiles. After a few minutes, the seizure subsided. I crawled into bed. When my parents came home, I began to explain what happened. But as I spoke, they were distracted by the sight of my tongue. The lower half was bloody and torn.

Dr. Dobbins raised my Dilantin level.

On August 17, 2002, I had my third grand mal while heading to the India Day celebration at Manhattan's Madison Square Park. We were midway there when the death scent hit me. I screamed to my friend Pablo, a Brazilian immigrant whose English was nearly nonexistent, to hail a cab. He couldn't translate fast enough. I was spasming on cold concrete once again.

But once again I learned how wonderful New Yorkers could be. A woman in her late fifties became my Mother Teresa. She squatted by me and gently rubbed ice cubes on my sweating, burning forehead. She also caressed my head, chanting over and over, "Don't worry about anything. God is with you. Everything will be fine."

I must have lost consciousness, because when I came to, the woman had been replaced by a cop. He offered to take me to the hospital, but I firmly declined. I asked him, instead, to hail me a cab.

I thought it was best to try another doctor. Dr. Dobbins recommended Dr. Clark, an epileptologist at a nearby hospital. We were told he was considered one of the best on the East Coast. We had nothing to lose. We gave him a try.

Dr. Clark was a superstar in the epileptology game, and looked the part. A man in his forties with a shiny ivory smile, he was tall and lean, with short, thick side-parted black hair, handsome, like a news anchorman come to life. Ordinarily, it took six months to get an appointment with him, but Dr. Dobbins helped speed up the process. I had my first meeting with him within two months.

Dr. Clark worked at a famous hospital in New York City. In his room, there was his epileptology posse: one student and two assistants. This guy was the shizzle. After studying my X-rays, he spoke to me and my parents, declaring with confidence, "There is a simple solution."

We were delighted and leaned closer.

"A lobotomy."

At that moment, I think the three of us collectively vomited inside our mouths.

"It's not as bad as it sounds," he said, and then noticed our sick-green faces. He lifted the X-ray so we could all see it.

"I hope you didn't think I said 'lobotomy.' I said 'lobectomy.' Quite different from a lobotomy. As you can see here, the culprit is the AVM scar. It is sitting on the occipital lobe. That lobe is destroyed anyway, so we can just get rid of it."

We were following him so far.

"Without the lobe, there'll be no scar. And without the scar, there is little chance that Ashok will continue having seizures."

We didn't want to follow him further.

"It would be a quick surgery. He'd only have to be in the hospital for four weeks."

My parents said we needed to discuss it. Dr. Clark suggested I check into the hospital anyway for a three-night stay, so he could fully check my brainwaves and classify my type of epilepsy. But I was so disturbed by the thought of the lobotomy, or lobectomy, or whatever he called it, that I never went back. I felt like telling him that my skull was not a jar of jelly that doctors could keep opening and closing at will, taking scoopfuls as they chose.

Time to find another doctor.

One of Mom's acquaintances, whose cousin had epilepsy, informed us about Dr. Jorgen. She said he was well-respected, although he wasn't mentioned in any of my growing collection of epilepsy books. Still, we gave him a shot.

A short, pale-skinned, and slender white man, he was in his fifties, with a stony face and a grim silver goatee. The first time we met him, I told Dr. Jorgen of Dr. Clark's lobectomy plans and he laughed. That was reassuring. He said it was a monstrous idea that would only cause more brain damage. He said he would offer effective treatment without cutting into my brain again. The first step, he said, was some in-hospital testing. He promised that all we would need was a high amount of a drug named Trileptal.

Dr. Jorgen's hospital was a shoddy space in New Jersey. The electrodes to my head were tied incorrectly and my tube connecting me to the monitoring device was too short; I couldn't even make it to the bathroom without nurse assistance.

The goal of the stay was to give me a seizure, so they could monitor it. They did everything they could to provoke it: make me hyperventilate, lose sleep, look at swirling lights. It wasn't happening.

On the fourth day, the nurses announced that I was to be discharged. They unplugged all eleven electrodes from my head. (Hurt like a mutha.) Then they had to strip the glue from my hair. I was unhooked from the monitoring tubes and brought to the shower, where I washed all the crap from my arms. Just as I was finishing, one of the nurses came in, panicked. It wasn't time for me to go, someone had made a mistake. I was rushed out of the shower and got plugged in and glued up all over again.

Ultimately, I never had a seizure in the hospital. They had nothing to observe.

Upon release, I was given Trileptal to take.

Dr. Jorgen had said this was the wonder drug, so I had bright hopes. Two days after being discharged, I had a complex partial seizure, in which I lost consciousness for a brief moment. It was not on the scale of a grand mal, but intrusive anyway. I still had to smell the fucking aura.

I called Dr. Jorgen right away and spoke with his second-in-charge, a woman named Lily, who was nowhere as dainty as her name might indicate. Despite my insistence that the Trileptal was horrible, making me sluggish, nauseous, and drowsy, Dr. Jorgen—through Lily—insisted I keep taking it.

Then came another seizure. I was in the car with Dad at the time. This seizure was a small one in which my head slumped back and drool seeped out of my mouth. Dad, unversed in caring for epileptics, shoved a water bottle in my mouth, a potentially fatal move.

After that I started doing more research on Dr. Jorgen, but could find no information on him anywhere, from medical journals to the Internet. However, my exhaustive research helped me come to better understand the nature of epilepsy. Doctors weren't the problem, it was the drugs, which were totally trial-and-error. If no seizure occurs, the drug dosage works. If one does, the drug dosage—or most likely, the drug itself—needs to be changed.

As a result, I didn't hate the doctors; I hated the way I was treated.

Then I suffered the very worst epileptic seizure of my life. It started June 25, 2003, at 5 p.m. I was supposed to see a movie with a friend, but I felt sick and stayed in my apartment.

The nightmare started. I smelled the aura; death was on me again. But this time it felt stronger than before. It seeped into every corner of my body. I started flailing and began chewing on my tongue until it bled. The aura had become the sphere in which I lived.

The electricity was so ferocious that my body started bouncing from one room to the other, bruising my arms, legs, and shoulders. I danced like an electrocuted marionette for ten minutes. And suddenly, it was over. I fell hard on the rug in my living room, lifted myself up to all fours and crawled to the bedroom.

Many minutes passed. I was first aware of a severe stench which nipped at hairs inside my nostrils. I turned my head on the pillow, but couldn't escape it. Then I started to choke and suddenly opened my eyes.

Shit was everywhere, as if I had finger-painted with it on the walls and floors. So was blood. During my hellish seizure, I had excreted and bled throughout the apartment. My body was bruised and bloody all over, from my legs to arms, from shoulders to back.

Luckily, my head was unscathed. I knew that God was watching over me. While my body had been flung around, my head could have easily hit the exposed brick wall and I would have been dead.

As I surveyed the destruction, I sobbed. Multiple thoughts—terrified and horrified—were running through my mind.

Look at the shit.

Blood everywhere.

The beige carpet has brown and red pools all over.

It's ruined.

I'm ruined.

I called Mom and Dad. They drove all the way from New Jersey, sped through the Holland Tunnel, and picked me up at the apartment. They brought me back to New Jersey. The next day I called Dr. Jorgen and left a message on his voice mail. I called again. No response—not even from Lily.

A week later Dr. Jorgen finally called, and invited us to his office. As I described the entire shitty, bloody, nightmarish incident, he listened quietly. Then he spoke.

"Let me ask you something, Mr. and Mrs. Rajamani. Don't you strictly watch over his pill intake?"

"Of course we do," Mom said, puzzled.

"Yet it's obvious he didn't take his medicine for this massive seizure to happen."

"I took the medicine," I said, as calmly as I could.

He just glared at me.

"I took the medicine," I repeated.

"Then there can be only one reason," he said. "Ashok, did you drink anything that day?"

"I might have had two or three glasses of water."

"There's your problem."

My parents and I looked at him blankly.

"You drank too much water," he said smugly. "You should never drink that much water when you have epilepsy."

All three of us dove in, yelling at Dr. Jorgen, accusing him of negligence and questioning his credentials. His face remained impassive as we hammered away. When we had exhausted ourselves, he stated authoritatively that he was a doctor and we weren't.

We had had enough of Dr. Jorgen. We walked out.

So Trileptal might not have been the ideal drug for me. But Dr. Jorgen should have at least recognized that. Or even better, he should have prescribed a different drug so that I would never again be forced to give my apartment a complete makeover.

As soon as I recovered from the seizure setback, I made an appointment with a new epileptologist. Dr. Feinberg kept hours at a prestigious hospital in Manhattan. He had a kind, reassuring smile and short, floppy blond-brown hair that fell down over his eyebrows. On my first visit, July 7, 2003, I told him my entire wretched epilepsy history. He listened carefully and prescribed a drug named Lamictal. I was struck by his laid-back style. Perhaps he meant to soothe his patients. Worked for me.

After our first meeting, however, I had a seizure that both shocked and scared me.

That morning I woke up around 11 a.m., later than usual. When I went to the bathroom to brush my teeth, my mouth felt strange. I opened it before the mirror and saw that most of the surface of my tongue had been chewed off, blackened.

I had experienced a massive grand mal seizure in my sleep.

Feinberg was characteristically comforting. He clearly came from the glass-half-full school of epilepsy. His assessment? A seizure like that was good, he said, since I didn't even have to be awake for it.

That's my Feiny, I thought, smiling inwardly. Leave it to him to make a near-deadly incident—many folks with epilepsy actually die by seizing during their sleep—into a cutesy line about the virtue of unconscious epilepsy.

He increased my Lamictal dosage.

Blacked Out

On August 24, 2003, an electrical blackout spread from the Great Lakes region across the upper Northeast.

At the time, Mom and I were in the waiting room of my primary doctor's Manhattan office. She had driven in earlier that morning from New Jersey to join me for this routine checkup. The air conditioner quit, and it immediately grew sweltering where we were. We grumbled, assuming there had been an electrical outage, but having no idea how far the situation had spread.

I started to sweat and then worry. I was beginning to smell an aura. I told Mom I had to leave. She told me to stay put; since it was a doctor's office, it would be safer. However,

I had a serious issue: each time I felt an aura, I felt the need to run—to run home, to run upstairs, to run any place. Perhaps I thought that if I moved fast enough, I could run away from the seizure that was about to strike. And today I wanted to run home from the doctor's office, since my apartment building was only five blocks away.

We told the receptionist we were leaving and hurried out. We still hadn't realized that there was a total blackout in the city. People were emerging from every side street, most of them frantic and confused.

I told Mom I was getting sicker and that the aura was growing bigger.

Then it happened.

On the corner of Twenty-second Street and Eighth Avenue, I started convulsing violently, and headed into the street. Mom called for help from two burly men walking by, and they helped her pin me to the sidewalk.

Mom's car was in a parking garage on Eighteenth Street. Once the seizure had passed, we decided to flee Manhattan and head to Jersey. But the lot attendant refused to let us in, explaining that trying to navigate the place without electricity was dangerous. But when Mom and I both begged, explaining that I was very ill and had to leave as soon as possible, the man relented.

In the darkness, we climbed to the second-story level, found the car, and drove it out. We didn't get far. Before us, the streets had become one big parking lot. It was a sight worthy of the apocalypse: thousands of little cars and Range Rovers trying to flee the city.

Too late. Too late to turn back and wait until hell has cooled a little bit.

And so we moved along in bumper-to-bumper traffic, one inch at a time.

Twelve hours later, we arrived in New Jersey.

Days after the blackout, I returned to Dr. Laid-Back Feinberg. He upped the Lamictal yet again. The seizures were finally controlled after that.

Seizures are often dubbed "mini deaths," since they present complete malfunctions of the body's brainwaves and, consequently, all organs. And to think, I was under the impression that my brain bleed would be the last death I would ever face until my body had actually expired, once and for all. That AVM sure left a bunch of unexpected, nasty surprises in its wake.

There's a theory that St. Paul's vision at Damascus was, in fact, just a seizure. Paul, you go, boy.

Through the Looking Glass: 2003–Present

The Eyes Have It

"I can't see my nose!"

(what?)

"My teeth are covering my face!"

(what?)

"My body is smaller than my thumb!"

(what?)

I couldn't believe what was happening. Everything around me was distorted, especially my own body. I looked into the mirror and screamed. I had become a monster.

All this started one day when I was in New Jersey, and Mom was driving me to Target to find a cheap rug for my Manhattan apartment. It was September 27, 2003.

During the early evening drive, the burgundy autumn

sky was easing into a dark black haze, and as I rode along, I became repulsively immature, believing I was not getting enough regard now that my epilepsy finally had been controlled.

Everyone's ignoring you, you need to get a reaction. You need to scare Mom, right now, I thought.

Right off Exit 11 on the highway, I spoke.

"Mom!" I yelled. "Everything looks so tall and skinny! That building over there looks thin as a stick, and taller than the sky!"

"Stop trying to scare me," she said. "You're just trying to get attention. It's not working."

"I'm serious! That movie theater looks like the Empire State Building! So high up and so much like a stick." I chuckled to myself.

"Your joke is failing," she said dismissively.

Then something strange happened. Everything ceased to be a joke. What I had pretended was suddenly happening. Within a second, the joke did not fail. It had become real.

"Oh my God!" I yelled. I was terrified.

"What now?" my mother asked, yawning.

"Everything really *IS* tall and skinny! Oh Lord! I can't see right!"

When we reached the store, I ran up and down the aisles, hoping I could see normally again. The shelves and TVs and computers and CDs all looked tall and skinny, so I ran to the men's restroom, wanting to see my reflection.

My body in the glass was as distorted as the store's merchandise. No, that's not right. It was even worse.

Arms were reaching my knees.

Legs were near my neck.

My nose was invisible.

Eyes stretched over forehead.

I looked around the stalls and urinals. Everything appeared distorted. My world had become a series of carnival freak-house mirrors. I ran out of the bathroom, more frightened than before.

Mom scolded me. "Calm yourself! We're going back home, and everything will be okay."

As we reached the driveway, I remained scared. The house looked small.

I screamed upon entering my old bedroom.

My childhood stuffed animals were now taller than me.

The television was the size of a knitting needle.

But even more terrifying were the distortions around me. Mom looked like a ghoul, all big eyes, no nose, with legs reaching her chest, while I saw Dad's head become the size of a chick pea.

But nothing was as bad as what I saw in the mirror; it reflected the same monster from the store restroom.

Dad, hearing my shrieks of terror, called the hospital emergency room.

"Help, my son is seeing a distorted world," he told a doctor on call.

"Don't worry sir, it might be just the onset of a migraine. It happens. I suggest that tomorrow morning you take him for a CT scan just to be on the safe side."

Relieved, he hung up and told me not to worry.

"Everything will be fine, in the morning you will see fine."

I fell asleep, exhausted after my intense spell of screaming and crying. Sleep was turbulent, though, as I was too worried about my sight to relax, though still hoping that everything would be okay. As day broke, I opened my eyes, scared of what I would see. The world was different from the tall-skinny visions of the night before, because now everything looked fat, squat, and short. It felt like I was in a coffin, as the ceiling appeared to be just inches from my head.

I ran to the mirror. A brown guy the width of a truck and the height of a gnome stared back at me.

Breathing in, my body became tall. Breathing out, my body became short.

The distortions changed with exhaling and inhaling; everything was shifting with the rhythm of my breathing. I was going insane.

"Mom! Mom! I still can't see right!" I cried out.

My mother tried to console me: "We're going to the doctor and get the CT scan. It's probably nothing." I wasn't convinced.

We went to the hospital ER where they took a quick CT scan. The doctor came back with a placid grin.

"His brain is perfectly fine," he reported.

Mom smiled.

"But I do recommend you see your eye doctor, anyway."

As we turned to leave the hospital, the doctor added, "I don't think you should see any average eye doctor. You need to see a neuro-ophthalmologist."

Days later Mom and Dad took me to Dr. Damore.

"Ashok says he can't see right, that everything is tall and thin, or short and fat," Mom explained.

He gave me a complete eye checkup, testing everything.

"His eyes," he told us, "are perfectly healthy."

"That's great to hear, doctor. So do you have any idea what the problem is, then?" Dad said.

"I think you should see your epileptologist; I feel it has something to do with epilepsy."

Mom and Dad looked down at the floor, silent.

"His name is Feinberg, isn't it?" he asked.

So we went to Feiny, who gave us a diagnosis when we met him. Frightening, maybe, but a diagnosis nonetheless. Dr. Damore was right.

"It might be seizures," Dr. Feinberg said. "Although seizures typically only last for less than two minutes, this could be the intense type that lasts longer."

I was led to another room. A kind older lady wet my head, parted the hair in seven pieces, and glued ten thick, hard electrodes to my scalp, using special medical-industrial skull coagulant. After wrapping the bundle of electrodes in a long white head towel, she attached the lower portion of the cords, which hung from the pale cloth's end, into an iPod-size instrument with a small screen.

Then she returned me to Dr. Feinberg.

"With this," he said, "we can see his brain waves."

He attached a long black joystick to the computer with a long white cord.

He gave me this contraption, saying, "We can test for seizures during a twenty-four-hour span."

Looking directly at me, he continued: "I want you to press this button every time you have a distortion. With each click, a red dot will show on the gray screen."

Nodding, I stared at the unit. I took it home, my electrodes and head-wrap firmly in place.

But the distortions never stopped. In the mirror I saw limbs the size of redwood trees. When I looked at my bedroom door, I would wonder how to get through a hole the size of a needle.

Upon returning to the doctor, after my headgear was removed, we looked at the gray computer screen. It was hardly visible under all of the red dots.

The joystick had been pressed sixty-eight times within one day.

"I have good news," Feiny said with a smile. "These aren't

seizures, since his brain waves didn't change at all during the times he pressed the button."

We thanked him and left.

Reaching home, I ran to my bedroom on the second floor and looked into the long, full-length mirror. *Perhaps this had all just been a bad dream.*

Nope. There were the distortions, still looking back at me.

While my parents were happy to know that there was no neurological damage, I was terrified not knowing why I was seeing what I was seeing.

All of the doctors, all of the diagnoses—nothing seemed to help. The distortions continued.

The days became a never-ending torture. Finally I decided to look through Dad's old medical books hoping to find an answer.

And there it was: "Hysteria."

In the book, the first section discussed the early definition of the word from the "Joseph F. Smith Medical Library." I read the passage:

"Hysterical disorder occurs when a patient experiences physical symptoms that have a psychological, rather than an organic, cause; an histrionic personality disorder character-ized by excessive emotions, dramatics, and attention-seeking behavior."

Turning the page, I discovered that medical professionals

no longer used the term *hysteria*. The word, I read, harkened back two thousand years, to Greece, from *hystera,* the term for womb. It was considered a female disease, a hyper-sexualization of the uterus which caused a woman to go mad.

I felt a wonderful stir of recognition, except for the womb part, of course.

I was excited! This is what happened! *I joked about the buildings, freaked out, cried and yelled, and had a hysterical response!*

But instead of hysteria, these episodes were now universally labeled *conversion reactions,* pathological conditions and symptoms without discernible physical cause.

I went back to Dr. Damore and Dr. Feinberg to explain to each the conversion reaction possibility.

I genuinely believed I had found the name for my unnamed affliction.

All three uttered variations of the same song:

"The idea of conversion reaction is quack science."

"It's what we medical experts call fantasy; we prefer to deal with actual, organic, physiological solutions."

"Labeling an illness 'conversion reaction' is the easy way out, a default diagnosis."

The doctors' words were terrifying, since the men could find no other official medical reasons for my affliction.

After hearing me out, Dr. Damore offered a final solution.

"Ashok, this might be, er," he said, "something best handled by a doctor specializing in . . ." he stammered, "psychogenic matters."

His incoherence and reticence puzzled me. "Meaning?"

"You need to see a psychiatrist."

Guess Who's Psychotic?

Rather than being horrified that I was being thrown into the hands of a goddamn shrink, I was thrilled that I might get answers, that I might learn that these distortions were, in fact, mentally and not physically created.

So I went to the neuropsychiatrist Dr. Damore recommended, Dr. Gold.

I met him in an exclusive, very impressive high-rise in Manhattan's Upper West Side.

After exchanging the usual pleasantries, during which I helped him with the pronunciation of my name, he led me to his office. Interestingly spartan, the rectangular room housed one large beige sofa, a reclining black leather chair, and an even more comfy, bigger black leather chair. He immediately sat on the third seat. I situated myself on the smaller chair. It faced his left side, so I was able to get a good view of him.

I immediately liked the man, really liked him. I don't know why, but I did. Carefully looking at the square steel-framed clock, he started speaking to me.

"So, Ashok, what can I do for you?"

"Didn't Dr. Damore mention my problem to you?"

"Very briefly. Now tell me the issue, in detail."

I told him everything, right from the drive to Target, the day the distortions started, to my recent electrode event.

"So, we know that your epilepsy is probably not involved."

"Yes," I said. "That's my crisis. If not that, then what?"

"Give me specific descriptions of your distortions."

I did.

His pen was moving continuously in his small olive spiral notebook. I wanted to know what he was writing.

"It seems clear to me what the problem is," he said when I had finished my tale of lunacy.

I didn't think I had ever smiled so widely in my life.

"What is it?" I exclaimed. "I have been waiting to hear this since it all began."

His pale white face became stern.

"Ashok, you are psychotic."

My first impulse was to laugh, which I did.

"I'm serious," he continued. "These continual distortions you're having . . . are hallucinations. The hallmark of a psychotic."

I had been called psychotic before, but by friends and family in moments of irritation, never by a licensed professional. I gave an unexpected Valley Girl response: "No way!"

I expected him to give an equally Cali-surfer teen answer: "Way!"

Of course, he did not. Rather, he offered a detailed explanation.

"The hallucinations you are having are called 'abnormal realizations' or 'unnatural thoughts.' As you told me, your doctors have not found any physiological explanations. So although these distortions involve physical conditions, I think they are definitely psychogenically oriented."

I sat motionless as I listened. Not only had my brain exploded; now I was crazy, too.

"Ashok," he said, "these 'unnatural thoughts' can be healed by medication. Let me write you a prescription."

I saw him look at the clock. My twenty-five minutes were up. He would now need a check for one hundred fifty dollars on which Dad already signed his name.

I was impressed by his quick but troublesome diagnosis.

"Thank you doctor, I'll get the med."

"Fine. I'll see you in two weeks," he said with a smile. He wrote the appointment on his calendar as I left the office.

I took that drug, but not before I went online to check out what it was. I discovered that this was a heavy-duty medicine used for only one specific type of patient: schizophrenic psychotic.

The realization did not matter, though. I was so relieved he had prescribed a cure that I took the prescription to the nearest Duane Reade and purchased the medication immediately.

For the next two weeks, the distortions never stopped. But I did encounter new experiences: I could no longer sleep without sweat, no longer breathe without congestion, and no longer urinate without feeling fire.

Thankfully, on my next visit, Dr. Gold immediately stopped the treatment.

"Doctor I can't take this drug anymore," I said firmly.

"You won't have to."

I was surprised by his quick acquiescence.

"I have thought this over. You're not psychotic at all. True psychopaths believe their hallucinations. You don't believe your distortions really reflect the world. This just might be a case of strong depression."

So instead of the hardcore mind-altering pill, he prescribed the simple commonplace antidepressant standby, Prozac.

The short career of Ashok the Psychotic was ended.

Taking Prozac didn't really help with my vision though, as my distorted world continued to exist, slowly drowning me in an escalating fury of fear. I eventually stopped taking that medication, too.

The White Rabbit Fucks Me, Long and Hard

The vision distortion changed me completely—no more exercising, eating right, or socializing. I couldn't look at the distorted faces of people I cared for; I couldn't bear to see them as monsters. Every day when I woke up and saw the world as abnormally distorted, I felt my sanity escape me a little more. I was now starting to believe my self-diagnosis, regardless of what the doctors said. Womb or not, maybe I did have hysteria.

Most of my time was spent looking through books, magazines, and online to help me find the cause of the continuing nightmare.

Finally, during one of my interminable daily hunts through medical websites, I discovered the name of an ailment that mirrored my own problem: "Alice in Wonderland Syndrome."

Dubbed AIWS, it was a neurological condition that affected perception.

The sufferer would see and feel everything in the wrong sizes. The syndrome was named because of its symptoms' correlation to the changes in size and shape that plagued Alice in Lewis Carroll's 1865 novel *Alice in Wonderland*. The site even said that the syndrome, in fact, often perfectly matched the original illustrations of the book.

It was an extremely rare condition that most doctors wouldn't even acknowledge.

Scholars, the site continued, speculated that Lewis Carroll may have been afflicted himself, since he suffered from migraine headaches. As she was Mr. Carroll's creation, Alice had to suffer the same fate of distortion when she reached Wonderland.

Confused, I remembered reading that Alice's hallucinations came from nibbling mushrooms, and that when she finally did battle with the Queen of Hearts she was allowed to escape Wonderland and leave the Walrus and the Mad Hatter behind. And best of all, she would never have to experience shape-shift again.

But as for myself, there was no Queen of Hearts to defeat, no Mad Hatter to meet, and no mushrooms to eat.

So how could I escape?

I sobbed in front of the computer screen, wondering how, and why, I ever met the goddamn White Rabbit in the first place.

Just as I suspected, my various doctors dismissed my ideas about AIWS, as well. Alice's wonderland, they told me, was for literature alone, not for reality. But later that week, when I returned to live in Manhattan, my eyes still belonged to Miss Alice.

Hermit Spiral: 2004

Monotype

Back in my apartment, my world was shrinking a little bit more every day. I spent most of my time inside my home. Yet even before the distortions, I had slowly begun veering away from contact with society.

I didn't have many friends and acquaintances even before the bleed, but I was confident my two closest buddies would be there for me: Zarina, who went by the name "Z," a tall Lebanese girl who had come to America for her education, and Jorge, a chubby Nuyorican whose humor got me through college. Unfortunately, it turned out I was wrong about their love for me.

They had been a wonderful support for my family during my hospitalization, but once I was released, everything changed. Z became a Tragedy Queen, thriving on my health issues. "I can tell you're not feeling well and it brings tears to my eyes," she said once.

At the time, I had just eaten a delicious Italian lunch and couldn't have felt better.

She offered to help me walk, although I didn't need help. I once overheard her mournfully tell her friends that she was busy caring for an aneurysm patient. After three months of Z's martyrdom, I said good-bye.

Good-time guy Jorge was a lot of fun. But the problem was that all of his rampaging involved liquor, and I no longer drank. One day he pleaded that he missed his old drinking buddy. He needed him back. But I wasn't going to drink again and risk killing myself. He still loved me, he insisted, but drinking took precedence. So Jorge said good-bye.

With effort, I was able to move on.

But it was my forced descent into Wonderland—the White Rabbit's vicious abduction of me—that plunged me into complete isolation. There was only one good development in all this: the distortions became limited just to the lengthening or widening of objects and people. No more bizarre distortions when I looked at my own body.

Still, the existent distortions caged me inside a dungeon I loathed. The utter loneliness began to choke me, and I couldn't breathe. When I was working in public relations, and was constantly around people, I believed that life would be better if I could have time just for myself. Like a virgin in bed with a whore, I had no idea what I was in for.

Being by oneself, I realized, was the cruelest possible condition. Especially in a place like New York City, where nobody ever smiles at another person, aside from those they know.

I forced myself to go out, maneuvering through the city streets alone. With daylight as my companion, I traveled alone to parks, movies, museums, and malls. Walking solo among others, I noticed my loneliness more keenly. Everyone else seemed paired off, talking and laughing while surrounded by coworkers, friends, and lovers.

Mom's Tears Return

Mom was right about the blame game she had predicted.

In the height of my loneliness-hopelessness period, I confronted her. We were both in the living room in the Jersey home, watching a *Nanny* rerun. As the episode broke for commercials, I looked up at her.

"I can't believe how awful life is," I moaned. "You did this!"

She gaped at me. "What are you talking about?"

"You gave me that filthy AVM. Because of you, I'm half-blind. And because of you, I have epilepsy."

"I knew you would say this to me," she said calmly. "Fine, I take the blame."

Unsatisfied with her response, I kept on. "With your diseased uterus, you did this!"

That comment earned me the reaction I wanted.

She started crying.

I was happy to see her suffer. "Good, cry! Maybe for one second you can feel the pain I will have to go through for the rest of my life."

She covered her face in her hands, sobbing.

"You are evil, destroying your own child."

Later that week, I came to my senses and begged for her forgiveness, sending her flowers, chocolates, and a Hallmark card of penitence.

Over an emotional phone call, she said she understood my sorrow, and welcomingly accepted my apology.

But I knew that she would never, ever get over what I had said to her. How could she? After all, at that moment, part of me had meant every word I said.

Sitting with the Old Man and Eating Soup with Streisand

Like vampires, we reluctant loners were brethren, connected by the bitter sadness of our unfulfilled lives. I was now able to hone in on lonely people more easily. One time, I wandered into a nameless Chelsea park. It was full of young parents and their children, playing, dancing, and simply enjoying their time together. I started to cry. I looked up and noticed an old man next to me. He looked at me in recognition. I looked back at him, a possible vision of my future, and I cried some more.

This is how my nonsocial life evolved. On weekends, I would go to my folks' home in New Jersey, where I did nothing except occasionally watch TV. PBS had some good British comedies on Saturday nights for people with nowhere to go. But on weekdays, back at home in my apartment in New York, this is what my datebook—if I had had a datebook—would have looked like:

8–11 a.m.

Sleep.

11 a.m.

Watch either *The View* or *The Price Is Right.* (I loved Bob Barker, that silver-headed charmer.)

12 a.m.

Eat breakfast of Special K in a bowl of orange juice.

12:30 p.m.

Watch *Who Wants To Be a Millionaire,* the palatable version starring Meredith Vieira.

1 p.m.

Watch *MAD TV.*

2–3 p.m.

Write a bit, go on Internet, look at E! Online.

3–4 p.m.

Walk around Manhattan. (No set pattern: some days, East

Village, others, Midtown. I probably saw every section of the damn island.)

5–7 p.m.

Job hunt.

7–8 p.m.

Nap time.

8–10 p.m.

Lupper. (I never woke early enough for three meals, so I had two: breakfast and a combo of lunch and supper, which I called lupper.)

11 p.m.–3 a.m.

Surf the net. Aimlessly.

Rinse. Repeat. Ad nauseam.

The highlight of the day—hell, any day—was lupper. Even though I had a kitchen in my cramped apartment, I never cooked. I just ordered takeout from trashy ethnic restaurants. Indian, Mexican, Italian, you name it. As long as it was cheap and greasy, it was lupper.

One day, I finally summoned the courage to actually eat out. I found my way to the Vietnamese-soup restaurant next door. The experience was surprisingly pleasant. This was a habit I wanted to continue. It gave me a much-needed sense of connectedness to the outside world.

There I met Gilda.

Gilda was my invented name for the lady sitting two tables

away. She came there every Saturday night. Her necklace exposed the Star of David, and she seemed to be in her early seventies.

Gilda wore at least five layers of cosmetics on her aged face. Her lips were painted far beyond her natural line. More strikingly, though, Gilda wore red, sequined evening dresses.

Obviously, her only venture into the land of the living was a Saturday night dinner. She probably spent the whole week planning for it.

During the three weeks I spent in that restaurant, I watched her every Saturday.

One night I felt fearless. After slurping down my egg-noodle soup, I went over to her table, and we exchanged names. Her real name was Lorna. Pretty close to Gilda. I was pleased with my psychic ability.

"Lorna, you must really love this place. I see you here often."

"They know me here," she said defensively. "Feels good."

"But I bet you also love the food."

"Food's okay. But leaving my place is even better. It's a cramped studio on Fourteenth Street."

"It must be a bad apartment, I guess." I smiled at her, and then asked with a laugh, "That's the city for you, huh?"

"Actually, it's not too bad. Young man, would you like to visit for dinner sometime?"

I then recognized how devastating loneliness would

become as the years went on. But would I want to be her dining companion? Sure, it's sexy for a young man to be with an older woman. But would it be sexy if she's an old Jewish white woman and he's a twentysomething Hindu brown man? How would it look for a geriatric Barbra Streisand and a young Mahatma Gandhi to go from dinner to the bedroom, to enjoy a sweaty, raunchy kink-o-rama?

I shook the gross image from my head. I felt dirty. I told Lorna I wasn't sure if I could come for dinner and that I'd let her know. Obviously, it wasn't the possibility of future kink that freaked me out. It was the possibility that, with my continuing solitude and loneliness, I was quickly becoming her. She gave me her number, a look of excitement on her face.

I never called her.

Forgive me, Lorna.

Lazarusness: 2004–Present

Shark

My sadness in my loneliness was gradually escalating into heightened self-pity and full-blown envy. I realized that I had been staying in the same place in life while everyone was moving on. Prakash may have altered his world during my hospitalization for those few months in 2000, but his life never stopped after that. He strengthened his new marriage, received his MBA, joined a worldwide restaurant corporation, and started his own realty business.

Jorge received huge promotions in his marketing company and had become a junior vice president. Z moved to Paris, and was getting married. My former college buddy Luis had become a high school calculus teacher and was now heading to Oxford. Moriyama, an obese old acquaintance and a self-proclaimed fashionista, had started an e-commerce company devoted to origami with his partner, Aaron. It had become massively successful.

Their happiness increased my nausea. Who the hell were they to succeed? I was the smart one, the creative one, the ambitious one.

Jealously toward my peers was nothing. I had even greater anger towards my dad. As a senior auditor for a worldwide pharmaceutical firm, he traveled internationally and inspected plants. While I was in recovery, Dad had traveled ten times, to Europe, Asia, Australia. Every time he went to the airport, I felt like screaming with angry jealousy. Here I was, stuck in my New York City apartment or in New Jersey, sitting in front of a TV.

I was immobile, while everybody in my life seemed to be moving forward.

I once heard that a shark has to keep moving underwater to live. If he stops and stays where he is, he dies.

I felt like I was dying. Fortunately, I realized I didn't want to.

Luckily, the burden of visual distortions was decreasing; I refused to pay attention to them, thereby stripping myself of my daily experience with them. While I continued noticing, intermittently, elongated or squat visions, I stopped being horrified by them.

Letter to Prakash

I often wondered how to possibly confess my rippling emotions to the primary blood-tie, who was born without defect:
my savior, my rival, my brother.

(First draft of a letter)

Dear Prakash,

Let's face it. I'm jealous of you.

Dammit. You did not get a birth defect, although we came
from the same womb. You have your full sight.

Dammit. You never have to fear seizures.

Dammit. You went to business school after my hospitalization and received your MBA from Wharton.

Dammit. After my hemorrhage, you continued to move
ahead in your life and your career.

Dammit. You created two real estate businesses and
scored a senior-level position in a major global hotel
corporation.

Dammit. You're happily married with a beautiful
home. Dammit, dammit. You have a million friends.
Dammit. Dammit.

You have a life.

I have none of these things. Well, I have a life. I lost it and
regained it. The only problem is, I'm not living it.

(Second draft)

Dear Prakash,

I beg your forgiveness. And Karmen's. I ruined your wedding day, the most special day of your life.

I ruined your reception; you never had that important first dance with Mom. I ruined the joy you were supposed to feel altogether.

(Third draft)

Dear Prakash,

Thank you for always singing the theme to *Good Times* while I was in my hospital bed.

(Final draft)

Dear Prakash,

Thank you for being there when I needed you the most. Everytime I look at you, I feel joy and gratitude. At the same time, I can't look at you without feeling despair and jealousy. I hope, one day, I can look at you without having any mixed feelings.

Understanding My Ticking Time Bomb

My mental correspondence with Prakash did nothing to alter the intensity of my jumbled feelings, nor the intensity of my sadness and isolation. I decided the only way to begin dealing with the situation was to find out, once and for all,

all about the culprit behind everything: my AVM. Because of the horror of the entire event, I had never done really intense, independent research on my birth defect, instead relying on doctors and their informational pamphlets to explain everything. There were staples and screws and metal in my head, that I knew, but I still couldn't spell out what happened within my cranium, and now I pored through this literature as if I were hunting for timeshares. Clearly I didn't want to accept that I had been born with a murderous defect.

I previously had decided not to dwell on what caused my grief. Now, however, after nearly four years, after my hundreds of lonely days, and after my encounters with Lorna and the old man, I was prepared to face it all.

I found out what percentage of people are born with this congenital birth defect that had caused my brain to explode: less than one tenth of 1 percent of the population in the entire world. It can also occur, to a lesser degree, in other bodily sites, including the spinal cord.

The actual definition, according to America's leading governmental neuroscience organization, the National Institute of Neurological Disorders and Stroke (NINDS):

> *Arteriovenous malformations (AVMs) are defects of the circulatory system that are generally believed to arise during embryonic or fetal development. . . . They are comprised of snarled tangles of arteries and veins. Arteries carry oxygen-rich blood away from the heart to the body's cells; veins return*

oxygen-depleted blood to the lungs and heart. The absence of capillaries—small blood vessels that connect arteries to veins—creates a short-cut for blood to pass directly from arteries to veins. The presence of an AVM disrupts this vital cyclical process. Although AVMs can develop in many different sites, those located in the brain . . . can have especially widespread effects on the body. . . .

AVMs account for approximately 2 percent of all hemorrhagic strokes that occur each year. . . .

If a large enough volume of blood escapes from a ruptured AVM into the surrounding brain, the result can be a catastrophic stroke.

I flinched when I read the term "catastrophic stroke." It certainly was an apt definition for my brain's explosion.

Also, I discovered that AVMs are disorders within a bigger crisis known as traumatic brain injury, or TBI. The facts about TBI astonished me. A few statistics: Over 2 million Americans suffer TBIs yearly; 5.3 million Americans live with a disability caused by TBI; in the U.S. someone sustains a brain injury every fifteen seconds; TBI-related deaths exceed AIDS-associated deaths and affect more people annually than AIDS, breast cancer, and multiple sclerosis combined.

But TBI receives virtually no federal funding.

And, according to Brain Injury Association of America, one of the gravest consequences faced by all TBI survivors is: "Total isolation and disappearance of socialization."

This diagnosis not only described my situation. It explained it.

Lazarus

With better understanding of the world of brain injury, I was finally ready to follow my doctors' suggestions and attend the TBI support group, my new peer community. I quickly bonded with one member: an outspoken woman in her late fifties named Nancy. She came from Russia and had a Ph.D. in English from Harvard. A brilliant and funny lady, she was fully functional except for a severe lisp. Her brain injury occurred when she was fifteen. An already brilliant little girl, she had been playing with her younger siblings in a park when she fell from the monkey bars; her head landed right on the concrete. At the time, Nancy was diagnosed with a minor brain injury. But when she was thirty it was discovered that her frontal lobe had been torn in the fall. Still, when we met I was dumbfounded by her knowledge: she was well versed in literature and psychology, even enjoying reading Lacan every now and then. Nancy's level of intelligence showed me that brain injury doesn't automatically mean becoming stupid and inarticulate. It gave me hope that I could maintain my intelligence. Finally, I realized that my overwhelming jealousy and isolation were hiding an upsetting truth.

I had been lost on a desert island, and the mainland was far, far away. But unlike those folks stranded on *Gilligan's Island*, I had nobody with me, not even the Skipper. At least I had stopped feeling self-pity; I was now in a state of rage. The whole world around me seemed to be set on "play," while my life was on "pause." I wanted to unplug this DVD player. As a result I vented in meetings, ranting about jealousy. I noticed that many others were nodding their heads in agreement. The more I ranted, the more everyone articulated their own grievances, their own jealousies. I did try to help the other members, though. A young woman who was recovering from an aneurysm started crying about how she felt useless, how she was like a child again and had to start all over.

"It's a good thing," I cheerfully said, offering a ridiculously lame affirmation. "Think of us like a new fashion line—we're hip, modern, fresh!" To the people who could comprehend what I said, this comment drew mostly groans. At one specific meeting, Charles, the young man who had been gay-bashed into complete, irreparable brain damage, voiced his anger over an *All My Children* episode he had just seen. An actor named Marco Judson now had the role Charles had played years earlier: a hunky construction foreman who was having an affair with the neighbor next door, as well as with her daughter. "That was supposed to be me!" he yelled.

Kari, our beloved moderator, faced him like a patient schoolteacher. "Charles," she said, "that Marco guy might have the role, but he might have some problems you don't know about."

"You mean like a mansion and a playmate wife?" Charles said, astonishingly sharp.

Kari sighed. "Mansions and playmates come and go, Charles, they mean nothing. You know that."

Charles gave a weak smile.

"The main thing is, he looks like he's balding pretty bad."

Charles gave a not-so-weak smile.

After one meeting, I spoke to Kari. "Can you let me know what happened to Charles after his beating by the cop? Did he seek compensation?"

"Charles's family sued the New York City Police Department for over twenty thousand dollars."

"That's great to hear, at least something was done."

Uncharacteristically blunt, she responded, "They gave him a check for five hundred."

Even with the occasional good cheer—and somewhat forced rationalizations—of group, I knew one thing for sure: I would never truly believe that surviving my brain hemorrhage was some fantastic achievement. After all, I was devastated by the pain, the personality changes, the mental deficits, the loss of a former identity, and most severe, the murderous isolation. For the rest my life, I would feel like the science class earthworm. Like that worm, my body and my being might have regenerated, but I would never be entirely whole, and would remain only a portion of what I once was.

Most group meetings would end with Kari giving us her "don't compare apples to oranges" spiel. If a brain injury survivor should compare herself to anybody, it should be to another brain patient, she cautioned. Once, Kari asked to speak to me privately after everyone left.

"You do realize how lucky you are, don't you?"

"Of course," I replied. "I even have 'survivor guilt' when I look at those poor people. I look relatively unscathed compared to them."

"Then why are you so upset? Look at them and realize how far you've come."

"But I see all my asshole friends making it big in the world, while I'm doing nothing."

As if talking to an infant, Kari said, "Ashok. I hate to put this to you, but you *were* crippled. You couldn't do anything at all. Look at you now."

The proverbial lightbulb finally popped on above my head. I *had* been crippled. She was right. I had come a long way since then.

And actually, my achievement was even greater than

Jorge's or Z's. I'd had to learn to speak. To walk. To think. And I did it all within four years. I hadn't merely pursued a new job—I had learned how to live again. None of my bitterness, resentment, anger, and jealousy could discount that. It took an underpaid social worker to teach me a truth that any moron on the street should be able to understand: I had learned how to live again.

That was more than enough.

Brain Karma: 1974– _____

God

I believe in God. There has to be a reason why I'm still here. Sure, the surgeons did a bang-up job in bringing me back to life. They inserted clips and resected veins and arteries in my skull. Nobody is dismissing their exceptional job. Peanut's not that dumb.

But, in the end, they were simply gas station attendants, while God was the fuel I needed to keep me alive.

To me, the Divine is beyond gender. Yet I now realize that God—male or female—holds an infinitely feminine power, though not in the way the West thinks of femininity, as a purely inactive, nurturing essence. Yes, that aspect is definitely present, but "female" power, described by us Hindus as *Shakti,* is ferocious, powerful, ruthless, and at times vengeful.

After my own hallucinogenic journey into "the liquid afterlife," God's cosmic uterus, I believe in the womanhood of God, represented by the sheer force of the hypnotic warrior-mother-goddess Kali, correlated with shakti. However, I couldn't have survived without the passivity of Lord Krishna, whose loving and warm sensuality embraces the nurturing side of both genders. Both worlds—the loving and the vengeful—assisted me in my path to resurrection.

Kali, her tongue ferociously extended, holds a sword. Krishna, the tender, affectionate deity, plays a melodious flute. The flute and the sword symbolize the two deities—the two aspects of God.

In my transformational journey, I veered back and forth from wielding the sword to playing the flute.

Moments of forcible rage swiftly changed to passive surrender. In the end, neither sword nor flute consumed me wholly. But the holy union of both saved me.

Teacher's Pet

Life is bondage. Everything we see around us is illusory, or *maya*. Reincarnation exists because we must return to goddamn earth again and again until we fully evolve—until we fully grasp the unreal nature of the material world. In other words, the body is a prison from which our souls must be freed.

After what happened to me, I've begun to understand.

Only when you witness your once-healthy mind and body

deteriorate do you realize that real life is unseen, beyond physical comprehension.

The whole thing is like high school; achieving ultimate consciousness and awareness is the equivalent of finally entering senior year. Spiritually, that's a level that usually takes numerous lifetimes to reach. Then, and only then, can we graduate and find salvation, or, as some might say, heaven. We can, at last, travel past even the Liquid Afterlife.

I don't know why I've been given a second chance on this Earth: to walk, talk, see, hear, and breathe. Having had the divine experience of swimming in God's womb, the experience of living after dying, I've worked hard to exist again, to move beyond the soul-and-body-scarring that began with one fateful orgasm.

God might be a strict, ass-kicking high school principal, but She's a fair grader.

Yet although I will never make valedictorian, I definitely won't flunk this time around, whether this journey ends tomorrow or two months or sixty years from now. I was granted access to enter the liquid afterlife, for at least a moment. So I think that I'll be moving up a rung in the next life, graduating to the next grade.

After all, I'm sure my brain's cum-triggered odyssey slash adventure slash nightmare slash resurrection has earned me, at the very least, a bucket-load of Bs in this lifetime.

And maybe even an A or two.

No Pity Required,
Just Fresh Breath: Present (I)

Horseshoe Souvenir

My craniotomy gave me a dubious and permanent gift: the horseshoe scar on the back of my damaged skull. Worst of all, everyone could see it but me.

Upon first returning to New Jersey after my hospitalization, my parents insisted that I leave the house occasionally to become accustomed to the outside world. We took tiny visits to nearby areas. As I walked with a cane, my body fell forward, or to the side. Sometimes Mom and Dad took me to parks. These outings were pretty uneventful, except for one time. We were sitting on a bench, when a young woman in velour track pants was passing by. She was walking her dog, but she stopped to look at me. Stare at me, actually. Irritated that she gaped at my head as if it were a Movie of the Week, I decided to shock her into running away.

I grabbed my crotch and yelled to my parents: "It still burns! I thought everything had cleared up, but Lord Almighty, it still burns!"

Dad and Mom laughed as the girl and her dog raced away.

The mall was worse. From the moment we got out of the car in the parking lot, I received stares: from adults, seniors, and of course, little kids.

I heard the same parent-child dialogue as I left the car, every single time. There were some variations, of course. But most were exactly the same.

"Momma, what's wrong with that man's head?"

"Don't stare, [insert child's name here]."

"Look, it's all cracked!"

"Shhh. Looks like something horrible happened to him. Poor man."

"His head doesn't look human!"

I was forced to hear this dialogue over and over, since the doctors had forbidden me from wearing hats for a while, all in the name of letting my skull "breathe."

There were, not surprisingly, other similar experiences: at a cosmetics counter where I'd gone with Mom, another at a movie Dad and I had gone to. Each time I felt both angry and sad, and even worse, very, very alone.

Brain Patients Just Wanna Have Fun

It took a long while, but I finally understood that my skull butchery was nothing to despise. Phil, my barber, was absolutely right when he told me that the marking on my head confirmed I was a survivor, and although he hadn't mentioned it, it also showed that I was blessed.

Discovering the power created by my scar, I opened my eyes to the conditions of all disabled, handicapped, sick, diseased folks in my walks though the streets of Manhattan.

Some were blind and wore sunglasses and walked with canes, some were in wheelchairs, some were amputees, some defaced by sarcoma.

Before my hemorrhage, I used to look at folks like these and think, *Oh, poor things*. But everything changed after I joined the club. Except that my situation was different. My numerous handicaps were internal. Unlike the others, with the exception of my scarred head, I looked perfectly fine to the world. When I bumped into somebody, or even tripped, folks just thought I was being rude or clumsy. Nobody guessed my brain was damaged.

When I tried to learn to walk properly again, it was hard work. When I tried to enter a room without knocking over objects or smashing my face against a wall, I had to work at it. I didn't want anyone to feel sorry for me; I just wanted to function as best I could.

Pity is useless. Pride is another issue altogether. When I see a blind man maneuvering through a subway station, I want to say to him, "Good for you! Enjoy the day!" Or, as the saying goes, "You better work, bitch!"

Handicapped men and women have enough to handle

without coping with condescension and unasked-for, piss-poor mercy doled out from the hands of anonymous passersby.

One single restaurant meal finally changed my mind entirely about the world of brain patients. I learned that we survivors are not only serious, dark martyrs who have lived through a nightmare and have, like Moses, found the Promised Land. I learned that we could have fun, too, just like everybody else. We could enjoy the big, wide, wacky world and be as ridiculous as our non-skull-scarred brethren. What magic to behold.

These realizations came when Nancy, from my support group, treated me to dinner after one of our meetings. Because it was in the height of a sticky New York City summer, we were skimpily dressed in tank tops and shorts. I could see her postmenopausal varicose veins; she could see my fur-infested arms. At just under six feet, Nancy was what one might call "statuesque." Although at five foot nine my height is probably considered average, in my mind, I've always felt too short. So, being arguably Napoleonic, I preferred to think of her as, simply, an Amazon. Nancy's long, gray-brown curly hair was pulled back in a ponytail, and her face was lightly painted. She wore appropriate-hued foundation to keep her pale skin dry, and decorated her mouth with subdued pink lip gloss. Quite foxy, actually. Nancy brought along Jim, not a member of the group, but a sixtysomething brain-injury survivor nonetheless, having suffered a stroke that left him partially paralyzed in his left arm. He was an elderly, plump white gentleman with gel-dried, side-parted silver hair. His chest was laden with a couple of tacky gold-plated necklaces, reminding me of those slick older men who produced movies in Hollywood's heyday.

Together, we looked like a trio from *Diff'rent Strokes* or *Webster:* a nice white couple with an adopted minority child.

Nancy, Jim, and I headed to a divey Burmese restaurant in Chinatown. As we sat down in the stuffy, windowless hole, we perused our ratty paper menus. After choosing our cheap meals, each under six bucks—quite a steal for Manhattan cuisine—we got to talking. Jim, it turned out, had indeed been a producer in the sixties. But not for movies. For Broadway musicals.

Let me explain here that brain damage affects victims in many different ways, and frequently manifests itself in what may seem to others as inappropriate and distorted behavior. For example, there is the anger that I felt, extreme anger, often directed toward anyone unfortunate enough to be nearby. That anger was most often sudden, quick to rise and just as quick to dissipate. Once your brain explodes, I suppose it's natural to feel a little bit of rage now and again.

Also characteristic—and this is by way of explaining and justifying, in part, the story that follows—is a lack of self-awareness and a lack of self-censorship in talking about our

own actions. My rudimentary grasp of these altered personality traits, though, did not prepare me for the shocking lack
of modesty that Nancy displayed in telling her story, a story
that, while stunning in the brilliant crudeness of its details,
was also revelatory to me in making me finally accept the fact
that pain and anger aside, there still was a potential world
of fun out there for me to enjoy in this life. Fun that could
involve breath mints, perhaps.

Conversation between the three of us, basically strangers, each of us damaged in some way by brain injury, had
been rather routine—until we started talking about sex. I
unintentionally sparked the discussion by telling them about
my fateful hotel orgasm. Soon my two dinner-mates began
sharing their sexual history with me.

Only I would get myself in this mess, I thought as the conversation took a decidedly graphic and raunchy turn.

The restaurant was noisy, with booming, wildly out-of-
place music playing over staticky speakers: Bon Jovi songs.
After Jim talked about his teenage masturbation sessions
(thankfully I went to the bathroom during most of his
speech), Nancy filled us in on a story that could be considered too cringeworthy for even a brain-damaged dinner
party like ours. Picture your mom telling this:

"The weirdest thing happened to me last month in Brooklyn," she said. "This guy I was dating went down on me."

"Then what happened?" I asked, straining to be polite.

Jim was obviously enraptured by her story, sitting with his mouth agape.

"After he got me all wet and juicy . . ."

I felt like cutting off my ears. Then burning them in a basement furnace.

". . . he decided to go further back, into my crack."

The waiter came by with complimentary orange slices. Having caught a part of the last comment, his face projected a blend of curiosity and the onset of nausea.

"And now here's the grossest part . . ."

What the fuck? There's an even grosser part?

"After ten minutes, he slowly moved up, higher and higher, and tried to kiss me! Could you imagine his breath?"

In addition to losing the superego—losing all self-censors and inhibitions—many brain patients lose some hearing. That meant Nancy was basically shouting this entire story, which, in a way, was fine given the loudness of the music.

In an appalling coincidence, however, the blaring music stopped abruptly, just as she finished saying "eating me out at both ends!"

Jon Bon Jovi's urgent big-hair vocals were now suddenly replaced by Nancy's big, big voice. Everybody heard, loudly and clearly, this lady roaring about getting her salad tossed.

The Burmese restaurant had become so unexpectedly quiet that the light jangle of Jim's golden bling sounded like vases shattering against a brick wall.

Being the mentally mishmashed folks we proudly were, we continued talking as if we had just been discussing a *Seinfeld* rerun. The crazy music started again, and sound filled the air once more. The restaurant soundtrack had replaced Bon Jovi with, insanely, the Supremes.

That was when we noticed a cute elderly East Asian man and woman sitting at a table next to us. They must have been in their seventies. I was so embarrassed. I couldn't believe we hadn't seen them earlier. At least we would have had a different conversation.

As we continued eating our orange slices, we were surprised as the sweet old lady leaned toward our table. With a look of bubbly excitement, she spoke to Nancy: "So then what happened? Did you kiss him or not?"

Becoming How the Brain
Became: Present (II)

Tenth Avenue

One balmy Sunday spring afternoon, I walked down Tenth Avenue and across Twentieth Street to the nearest Gristedes grocery store, desperately in need of my latest regular home cuisine: nonfat pineapple-flavored cottage cheese. I was wearing my typically nondescript, standard May wardrobe selection: plain white tee, khaki cargoes, and five-buck flip-flops. Walking past a rather empty intersection, I noticed a stolid thirtysomething lady pushing a young boy in a wheelchair. Looking to be maybe ten years old, he appeared severely developmentally disabled, head erratically jerking and cocking far to the right, wide grin contorting his mouth, and with glazed, empty eyes aiming toward the heavens. He looked bald in the sunlight, with his blond hair neatly shorn into a presummer crew cut.

As they passed by, I witnessed the most astounding thing. Above the headrest of his wheelchair, the back of the boy's nearly hairless head came into view.

It was completely scarred.

It looked like it was stitched together with patchy horsehide. It looked like it was a tic-tac-toe board. It looked like it had been destroyed.

I ran after them, suddenly intent on talking to them.

"Ma'am," I said to the woman. "Sorry to bother you, but can I please ask you a question?"

I didn't wait for a reply. "Did this child have brain surgery?"

She stared at me with a look of panic and irritation, as if I were a deranged terrorist attacker, or at worst a telemarketer. I couldn't tell if she felt anger, curiosity, surprise, or, most likely, a combo of all three.

"Who the hell are you, and why the hell do you care?" she said warily.

"My name is Ashok. It's just that I had brain surgery, too."

I could tell she didn't believe me, but she answered right away. "Yes, he did have that."

"Can I ask what was the reason for his surgery?" Whereas at first she looked defensive, she now seemed grateful, as if discussing the boy's situation, even to a complete stranger, brought her some relief. Perhaps, I thought, her friends and family avoided any discussion about the child's situation.

"Well, Ashok," she said (she pronounced it "choke," which was better than 98 percent of folks did), "I'm Sara, and this is my son Kevin."

"Hi, Kevin!" I boomed at the kid. "You having a good time?"

Of course, he said nothing.

I turned to Sara. "I'm really sorry to disturb you, though. You must be on your way somewhere, and here I am, bothering you."

"Not at all, we were just taking a leisurely walk. It's so nice out."

I gave her a reassuring smile.

"So I suppose I'll tell you what happened. I have nothing else to do anyway." She laughed.

I nodded slowly. "That's real nice of you, Sara."

She started speaking in a barely audible murmur. "Well, he had something called an AVM. It's a birth defect of screwed-up veins in the brain. He was getting headaches all the time, so the doctor tested him. Found out this AVM thing was the problem. So they did the surgery, took the thing out.

"The surgery made him paralyzed from the waist down. And he's been left completely retarded. But everyday I thank God that he survived . . ." Her quiet voice paused before continuing. ". . . And he is still here. My baby is alive. My Kevin is alive, alive, alive."

Sara began crying gently. She dried her tears with a tissue from her oversized handbag.

"He looks fantastic," I said.

"Thanks. He's getting better. He really is."

Her face suddenly hardened. "So what do you mean you had brain surgery, too? No you didn't. That's a disgusting thing to lie about."

"I'm serious," I said, as I turned my head around, carefully parting the hair on the back of my head, near my right ear, to reveal my once grotesque but now lucky horseshoe-shaped scar. "And I have something else surprising for you, Sara."

"I doubt it," she said. "The way you look is surprising enough."

Taking a deep breath, I spoke. "I had an AVM, too. That's the reason for my brain surgery."

"Oh my God!" she yelled, her eyes opening wide, wider than I thought possible, before she hugged me tightly. And then, a surprise high five. "You've got to be kidding me. I thought only one in a kazillion kids get that disgusting thing."

"Well, I suppose Kevin and I are among those lucky folks!" I said. "Remember, someone's gotta win a raffle or a state lottery or a Powerball, even though the odds are crazy, slim to none. But someone *always* wins. I guess Kevin and I won this specific lottery."

"I suppose. But I'm his mom. I want to kill myself for doing that to him."

Thinking of my own past adventures in blaming my mother, I said, "Stop thinking like that. You had no control over it. Like I said, someone's gotta win the lottery."

She continued dabbing her eyes with her Kleenex.

"Sara, don't worry. I promise you, he'll be okay. I, too, couldn't walk and my mental state was in tatters. Kevin will get better. Maybe not next week or next month, but it'll happen. I promise you. I'm doing great. So will he. Take my word."

Sara smiled through her tears. "Well, we should get going now," she said abruptly.

"Sure thing. Thanks so much for the talk. Bye guys."

"Thank you, Choke."

Looking at her boy one last time, I whispered quietly, only to myself, "You'll make it, Kevin."

I stood still as mother and son strolled past me, headed up the avenue. There was no exchange of numbers.

For some reason, just then the Burmese restaurant outing popped into my head. I couldn't help but think of Kevin, and my fellow brain-injury survivor-warriors around the world, specifically the little battle-scarred craniotomite girls and boys. Regardless of how altered their conditions might have become, they were still alive, in a world with so much joy for them to experience.

And so many of life's ridiculous wonders to look forward to.

I watched as Sara and Kevin turned a corner four blocks ahead of me. I didn't know where they went, just as I didn't know where I was headed.

Yes, my life has been restored, but what I am experiencing is not simply the refurbishing of my old existence. This is, in actuality, a brand new life. As much as I hate to admit it, a guy named Ashok, or perhaps I should say, Ashok 1.0, died on March 17, 2000. A long and difficult gestation followed, but Ashok 2.0 has risen, entering a land that, though familiar in many aspects, is unlike anything the first Ashok experienced before.

I am now calmer and ready for a wide-open future. Oddly enough, even though I face epilepsy and multiple functional deficits in my sight, hearing, and memory, I've become more at peace, finding a new kind of harmony with the world.

Of course, I never was, never am, and never will be a full-fledged "norm." I will always be an involuntary outsider. My attempts to symphonize the melodies of my circumstances, from snowy cornfields to icy urban sidewalks, have never succeeded. And I certainly have no delusions that everyone will view me with undiluted acceptance.

Even though the entire experience has raised my re-incarnation GPA closer to a 4.0, I'll always be confounded by the miracle of being granted two lives in this one Baby Buddha avatar. I dearly miss Ashok 1.0, with his holy-war-mongering, his unintentional arrogance, his liquid lunch-and-breakfast-and-dinner work ethic. The detonation of my brain, however, has thrust me into a freshly focused soul, one that realizes why creating publicity for a silly magazine means little, and why creating hope for anyone in a wheelchair means everything.

I loved that old guy profoundly, but I think I love this new fucker just as much.

Perhaps even more.

PRAKASH DRIVES ME back to my Manhattan apartment after I visit one of my countless doctors in New Jersey. It is an unnaturally humid autumn afternoon, with leaves looking as if they're falling not because of chilly winds, but from heat-stroked exhaustion.

The car radio is blasting forgettable yet addictive dance-pop tunes.

His wedding ring grazing the steering wheel of his aged Toyota Camry, Prakash tells me, "I still can't believe what happened to you."

Chuckling, he adds, "And you thought school was tough."

"True," I say, sounding far more solemn than I had intended.

"Hey Dumbass, you're going to have lots of problems because of all that metal in your head," he says.

"Like what, Numbnuts?"

"When you go to the beach, your head's gonna be surrounded by all the folks with mining detectors trying to find metal stuff in the sand!"

He laughs loudly, forming his own boisterous cheering squad.

His dorkiness, I realize with love and admiration, is fabulous, whereas mine, historically, is just plain embarrassing.

"You do know the Showtime at the Apollo audience would boo your ass off the stage, right?" I say.

"What are you talking about?" Prakash says loudly, deadpan and on cue. "I have a great sense of humor. That's my gift from God."

"Some gift," I respond, as the music thumps urgently.

His tired joke will probably flunk Comedy 101, but it jars me into thinking about my odyssey, and the horseshoe engraved between my ears.

My badge of honor. My unlikely badge of honor.

I hum to the swirling bubblegum beats that vibrate in the car. Glancing at the side-view mirror, I see my reflection, that man who was/is Ashok. He is smiling back at me. Even though the sun's filtered rays cast impenetrable black shadows, I can see that he is smiling back at me. Even though the car's speed creates vibrations that jar the mirrored surface, I can see that he is smiling back at me.

The brown guy in the mirror looks happy.

I gently caress my carved warrior skull as the car accelerates past a yellow light, grooving ahead toward the future.

Acknowledgments

I AM FOREVER INDEBTED to my amazing editor, Chuck Adams, whose guidance, wisdom, and enthusiasm made this book possible, from beginning to end. Chuck, it has been a privilege to work with you, and I thank you for taking a chance on this unknown, brain-damaged, Indian American redneck.

Thanks to the tribe:

Prakash: You were my first responder and savior. Your little brother loves you.

Mom: Words cannot express how much you mean to me. You never left my side, and I never could have survived without your encouragement, love, and strength. I'm truly blessed to have you as my mother.

Dad: Thank you for your unconditional love and support through everything; you're a wonderful father, and a wonderful man.

Puthucode Ramanan Uncle: You showed me the virtue of letting go.

Lakshmi: Love you, my precious niece.

Karmen: Thank you for being there for us.

Ramakrishna Parameshwar Aiyer: You were not only my grandfather, but my idol and inspiration.

Meenakshi Aiyer and Rajam Swamy, my spitfire grand-mothers: I'd like to think some part of your gorgeous fierce-ness rubbed off on me. And to every other departed elder of my family: I will always cherish you, and hope you're proud of me, wherever you are.

Thanks to the healers:

My neurologists; neurosurgical team; neuro-ophthalmologist; neuropsychologist; neuropsychopharmacologist; epileptol-ogist; otorhinolaryngologist; psychotherapist; infectious-disease doctors; cardiologists; hospital nurses in the inten-sive care units and neuro-critical care units; physical, visual, speech, cognitive, and occupational therapists; and medical advisors. Thank you all from the bottom of my heart.

Thanks to the team:

The Algonquin/Workman crew, namely Brunson Hoole, Kelly Bowen, Elisabeth Scharlatt, Bob Miller, and Chris Stamey; Emma Sweeney; Jeremy George; Thangam Aiyer; Kashmira Shah; Renu Shah; the Chinwalas; Pat Sajak; Fuaud

Yasin; Lennon Safe; Fred Guerriero; Penelope Franklin; Moko Hirayama; Sallie Randolph; Vanna White; Jay Blotcher; my educators at Avon Center School; and all the dear friends I've made as Ashok 1.0, and now as Ashok 2.0. Special thanks to Tom Dobbins and Timothy D. Bellavia.

I'D LIKE TO give a very personal tribute to my fellow AVM and brain surgery survivor-warriors, as well as to those who have bravely fought and overcome aneurysms, hemorrhages, strokes, and all forms of brain injury; to the visually handicapped; to those living with epilepsy; and to the courageous little Indian American boys or girls growing up in Small Town, USA, fighting for the correct pronunciations of their names. Rock on.

Above all, I salute my Highest Power, without whom I would not still be living and breathing. *Hari Bol. Om.*